Atlas and Manual of
CARDIOVASCULAR MULTIDETECTOR COMPUTED TOMOGRAPHY

Atlas and Manual of
CARDIOVASCULAR MULTIDETECTOR COMPUTED TOMOGRAPHY

Paul Schoenhagen MD FAHA

The Cleveland Clinic Foundation
Cleveland, Ohio

Richard D White MD FACC

Arthur E Stillman MD PhD

Sandra S Halliburton PhD

Foreword by

Michael T Modic MD FACR

Division of Radiology
The Cleveland Clinic Foundation
Cleveland, Ohio

Eric J Topol MD

Department of Cardiovascular Medicine
The Cleveland Clinic Foundation
Cleveland, Ohio

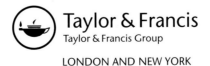

Taylor & Francis
Taylor & Francis Group

LONDON AND NEW YORK

© 2005 Taylor & Francis, an imprint of the Taylor & Francis Group

First published in the United Kingdom in 2005
by Taylor & Francis,
an imprint of the Taylor & Francis Group,
2 Park Square, Milton Park
Abingdon, Oxon OX14 4RN, UK

Tel.:   +44 (0) 20 7017 6000
Fax.:   +44 (0) 20 7017 6699
Email: info.medicine@tandf.co.uk
Website: http://www.tandf.co.uk/medicine

Although every effort has been made to ensure that all owners of copyright material have been acknowledged in this publication, we would be glad to acknowledge in subsequent reprints or editions any omissions brought to our attention.

British Library Cataloguing in Publication Data

Data available on application

Library of Congress Cataloging-in-Publication Data

Data available on application

ISBN 1-84214-302-6

Distributed in North and South America by

Taylor & Francis
2000 NW Corporate Blvd
Boca Raton, FL 33431, USA

Within Continental USA
Tel.: 800 272 7737; Fax.: 800 374 3401
Outside Continental USA
Tel.: 561 994 0555; Fax.: 561 361 6018
E-mail: orders@crcpress.com

Distributed in the rest of the world by
Thomson Publishing Services
Cheriton House
North Way
Andover, Hampshire SP10 5BE, UK
Tel.: +44 (0) 1264 332424
E-mail: salesorder.tandf@thomsonpublishingservices.co.uk

Composition by Parthenon Publishing
Printed and bound by T. G. Hostench S.A., Spain

Contents

Acknowledgement

We wish to acknowledge the technologists and nurses in the Radiology Department at the Cleveland Clinic Foundation.

List of authors

Paul Schoenhagen MD FAHA
Department of Radiology, Section of Cardiovascular
   Imaging
Department of Cardiovascular Medicine
The Cleveland Clinic Foundation
Cleveland, Ohio

Richard D White MD FACC
Department of Radiology and Cardiovascular
   Medicine
Clinical Director, Center for Integrated Non-Invasive
   Cardiovascular Imaging
The Cleveland Clinic Foundation
Cleveland, Ohio

Arthur E Stillman MD PhD
Department of Radiology, Section of Cardiovascular
   Imaging
The Cleveland Clinic Foundation
Cleveland, Ohio

Sandra S Halliburton PhD
Department of Radiology, Section of Cardiovascular
   Imaging
The Cleveland Clinic Foundation
Cleveland, Ohio

List of contributors

Stacie A Kuzmiak RT (R) CT
Department of Radiology, Section of Cardiovascular
    Imaging
The Cleveland Clinic Foundation
Cleveland, Ohio

E Murat Tuzcu MD FACC
Department of Cardiovascular Medicine,
Medical Director, Intravascular Ultrasound Core
    Laboratory
The Cleveland Clinic Foundation
Professor of Medicine,
Cleveland Clinic Lerner College of Medicine
Case Western Reserve University
Cleveland, Ohio

Steven E Nissen MD FACC
Department of Cardiovascular Medicine
Medical Director, Cleveland Clinic Cardiovascular
    Coordinating Center
The Cleveland Clinic Foundation
Cleveland, Ohio

Randolph M Setser DSc
Department of Radiology, Section of Cardiovascular
    Imaging
The Cleveland Clinic Foundation
Cleveland, Ohio

Joanie A Weaver RT (R) MR
Department of Radiology, Section of Cardiovascular
    Imaging
The Cleveland Clinic Foundation
Cleveland, Ohio

Timothy Crowe BS
Department of Cardiovascular Medicine
Technical Director Intravascular Ultrasound and
Angiography Core Laboratories
The Cleveland Clinic Foundation
Cleveland, Ohio

Editors' note

Cardiovascular computed tomography (CT) imaging is a relatively new and rapidly evolving diagnostic modality. Growing experience and advances in CT scanner technology constantly expand clinical applications.

This atlas provides comprehensive information about cardiovascular CT technology, imaging protocols and clinical indications. These are described by a team of authors including clinicians, CT technologists and imaging physicists. A comparison with other imaging modalities such as conventional angiography, intravascular ultrasound, magnetic resonance imaging and echocardiography allows understanding of the current strengths and limitations of CT in the assessment of specific clinical questions.

The majority of the images are acquired with 16-slice technology. However, the recent transition to scanners with more than 16 slices is reflected. The figure legends include parts of actual report text, allowing a guide to description of similar cases. The index refers to both the text and the images, providing easy access to the information.

Despite the extensive information collected in this book, it is important to emphasize that it is not intended to provide a systematic discussion of cardiovascular imaging. This atlas provides the reader with a guide to the performance and interpretation of cardiovascular CT based on a large number of selected clinical images.

The enclosed CD provides a number of movies which further illustrate selected findings with CT.

Foreword

Very rarely in medicine is there truly a revolutionary advance that has the capability of radical transformation of clinical practice. Now, with MDCT, it is entirely possible that diagnostic coronary angiography may be headed towards obsolescence over the years ahead. MDCT is truly a 'disruptive' technology. It challenges traditional models for how and by whom diagnostic evaluation of cardiac morphology and function, and, specifically coronary anatomy, is best carried out.

This advance in CT technology has had a paradoxical effect in both lowering and raising the skill set and knowledge threshold necessary to acquire and interpret advanced cardiac imaging. In select cases, cardiac and coronary anatomy can be depicted in minutes without resorting to cardiac catheterization. The acquisition itself and subsequent analysis and interpretation, however, are more complicated than initially perceived. Patient selection, individualized imaging protocol design, multiple-organ system assessment, pharmacology, radiation safety, post-processing and artifact recognition are interactive and critical factors in maximizing the impact of this exam on clinical decision making.

When new technology changes the nature of a service, challenges occur. The traditional approach to new technology is often specialty specific and overly influenced by the business model. Adoption and ownership often accrues to the specialty that accommodates more quickly, especially if it falls with in its sphere of expertise. However, when a disruptive technology, to be employed maximally, requires the skill sets of multiple specialties, then the practice models need to change to accommodate. This is not always easy with our traditional vertical silos of medical specialties but critical in the case of cardiac MDCT. True multidisciplinary teamwork is exemplified by this text and the example set by the authors in this regard is laudatory. The collaboration and synergy created by this group of cardiologists, radiologists, cardiothoracic surgeons and acquisition/post-processing basic scientists – and, perhaps as importantly, critics – has resulted in true innovation and adoption.

The challenges will continue. This technology is continuing to evolve with a half-life shorter that any other innovation in memory. As of this printing, 16-row CT is being quickly superseded by 40- and 64-row scanners. The 128- and 264-detector systems, multiple tubes, dual energy and more sophisticated post processing are just around the corner. Standardization and more turnkey examinations are sure to follow. Notwithstanding, the value of this text will survive for two important reasons. The first relates to the value of its content as an educational vehicle and introduction to the technology and cardiac diseases. The advances in the future will be one of degree rather than the quantum leap from the traditional that this text depicts. MDCT may be supplanted by advances in other areas of imaging technology or become part of other acquisition strategies as not only medical specialties but technologies combine. The second relates to its example of teamwork and sense of direction towards true multidisciplinary integration and collaboration. These challenges are best answered in a collaborative environment of discovery and this text exemplifies the synergy of what can be created by such a joint effort.

Without question, MDCT will be an important imaging technique of the future and we believe this *Atlas and Manual* will be a valuable resource for the burgeoning medical community who will be active in shaping its appropriate application.

Michael T Modic MD FACR
Chairman, Division of Radiology
The Cleveland Clinic Foundation
and Professor of Radiology
Cleveland Clinic Lerner College of Medicine
Cleveland, Ohio

Eric J Topol MD
Provost, Cleveland Clinic Lerner College of Medicine
Chief Academic Officer, Cleveland Clinic Foundation
Chairman, Department of Cardiovascular Medicine
Professor of Medicine and Genetics, CWRU
Cleveland, Ohio

Color section

The following figures are color versions of selected figures from the main body of the text.

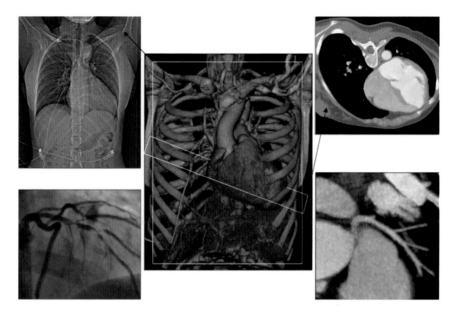

Figure 1   Planar versus tomographic imaging

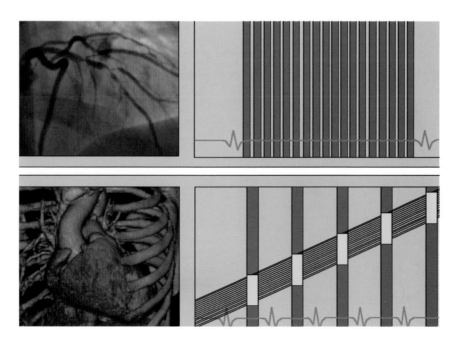

Figure 2   Image acquisition time

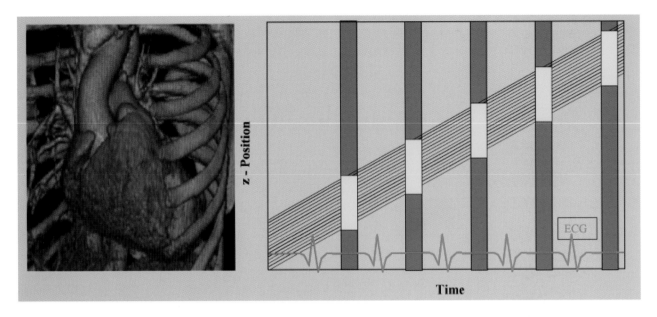

Figure 9   Volume coverage

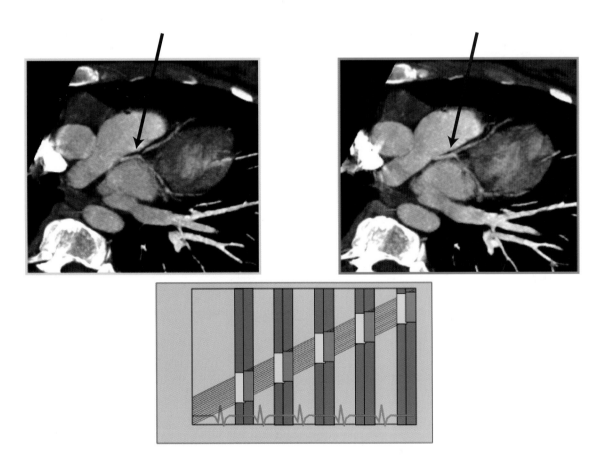

Figure 10   Reconstruction window: image quality

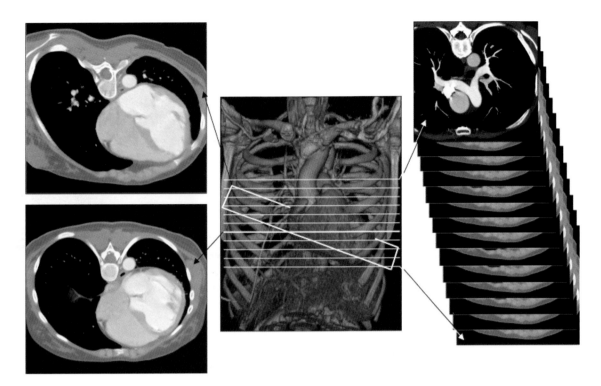

Figure 18 Axial and oblique images

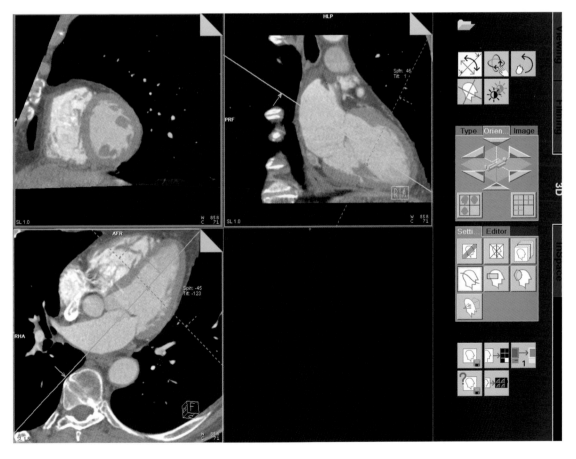

Figure 20   3-D workstation (1): oblique planes, left ventricle

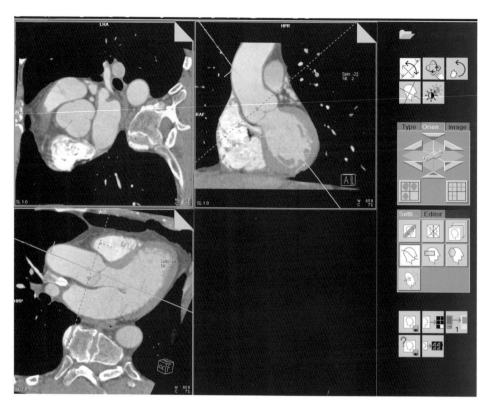

Figure 21   3-D workstation (2): oblique planes, aortic root

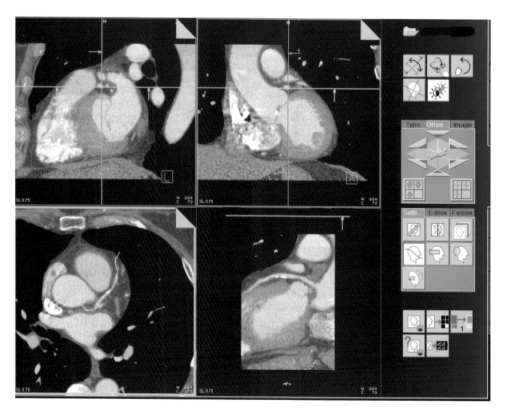

Figure 22   Curved 2-D reconstruction (1)

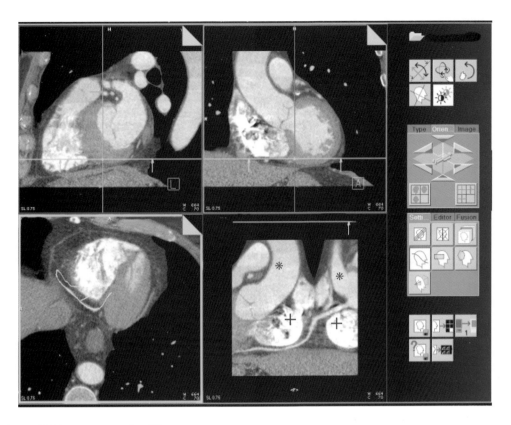

Figure 23   Curved 2-D reconstruction (2)

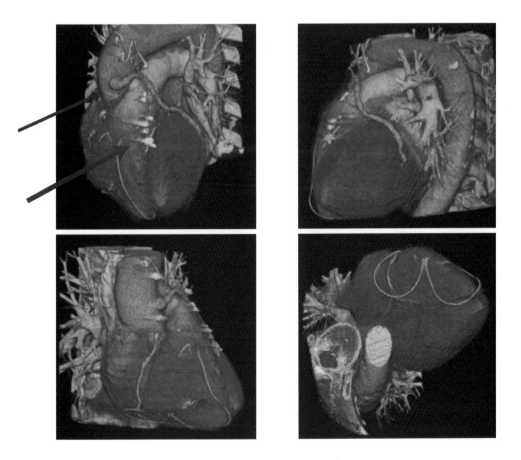

Figure 26   Color-coded VRI

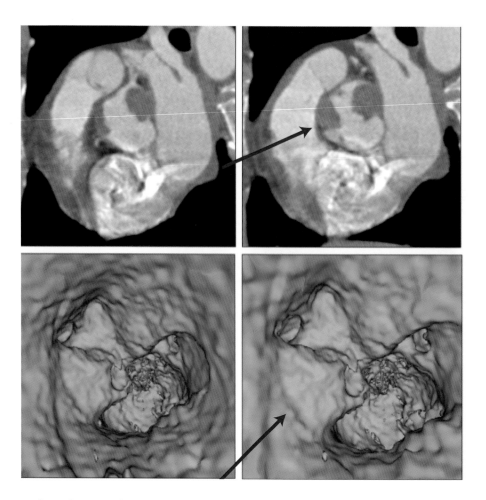

Figure 27 Perspective volume rendering

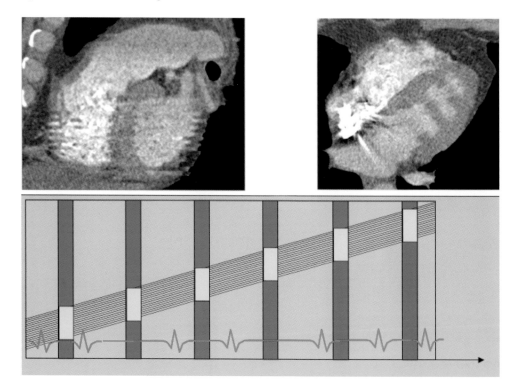

Figure 29 Arrhythmia artifact (1)

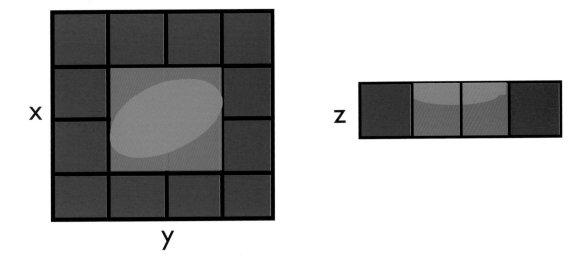

Figure 33   Partial volume averaging: blooming artifact

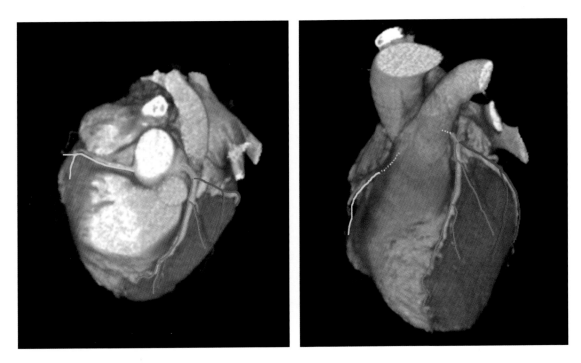

Figure 42   LAO view of coronary arteries

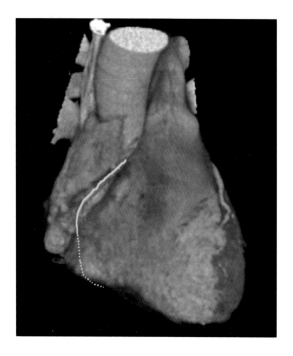
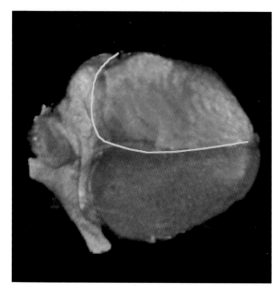

Figure 44 RAO view of coronary arteries

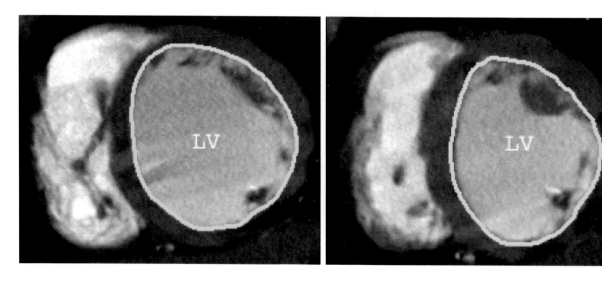

Figure 46 Left ventricular function

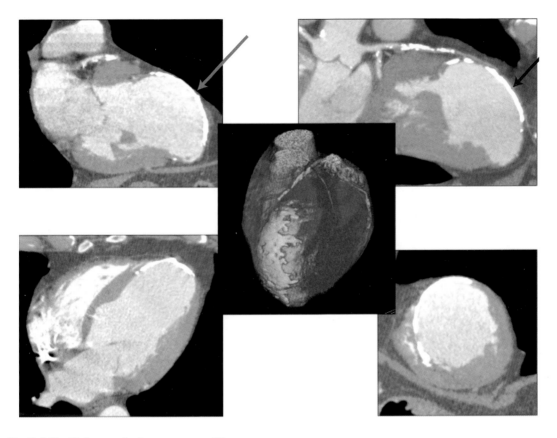

Figure 67 Calcified left ventricular aneurysm (1)

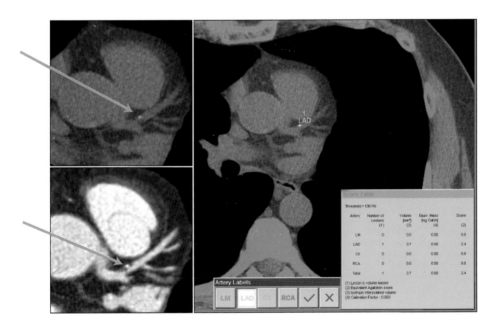

Figure 90 Calcium scoring

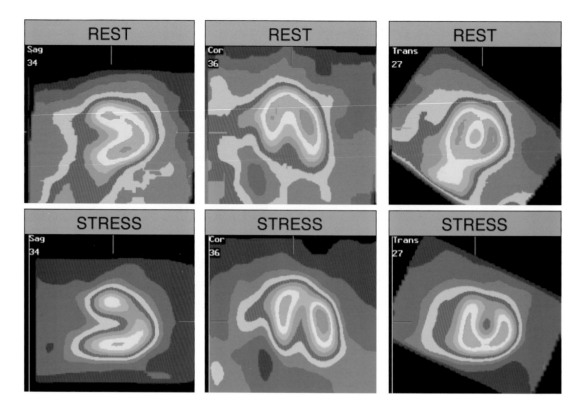

Figure 109   Significant luminal stenosis (2.5)

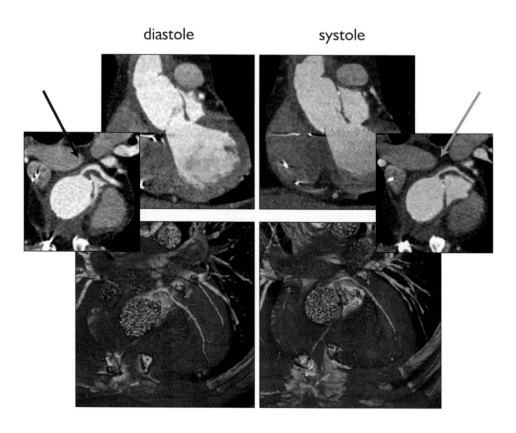

Figure 117   LV outflow tract pseudoaneurysm causing coronary compression (1.2)

diastole systole

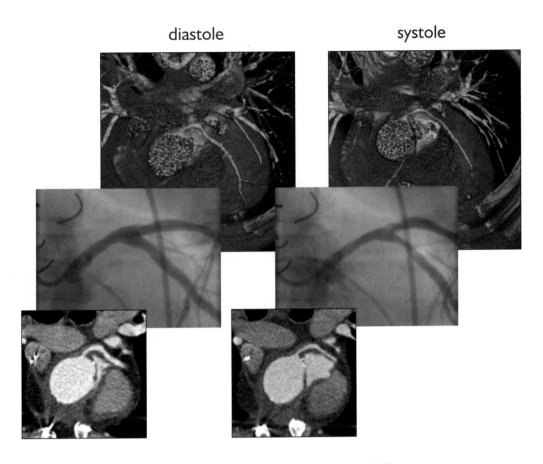

Figure 118 LV outflow tract pseudoaneurysm causing coronary compression (1.3)

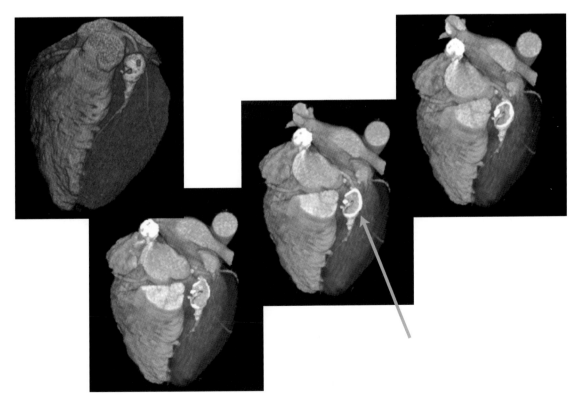

Figure 121 Left anterior descending coronary aneurysm (1.1)

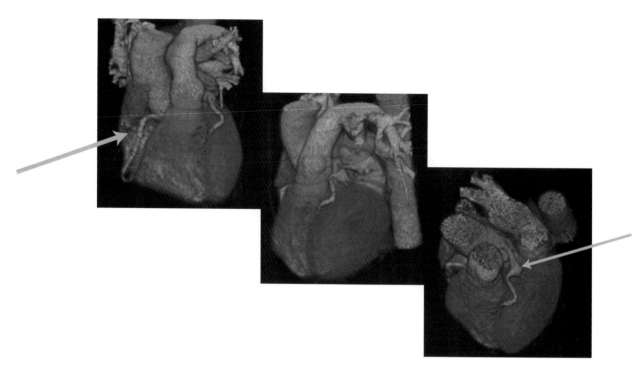

Figure 125   Diffuse coronary ectasia (1.1)

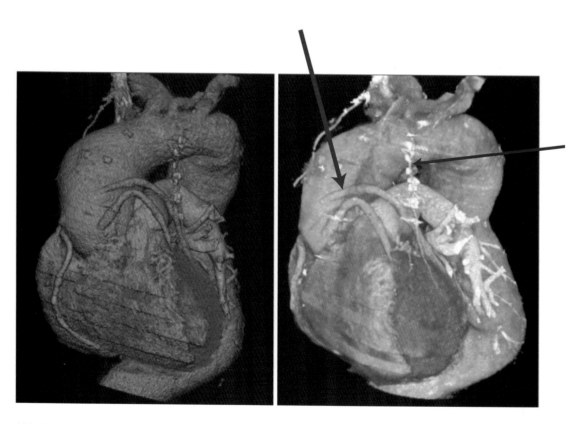

Figure 129   Bypass graft assessment (1.2)

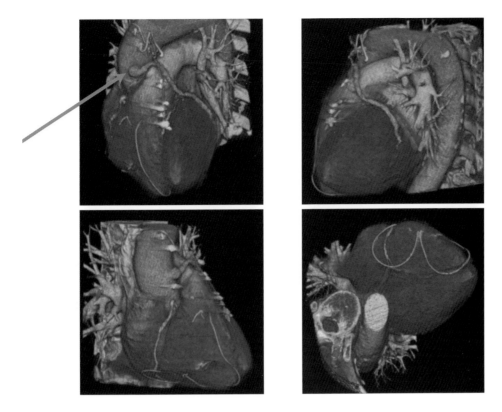

Figure 132 Stented bypass graft (1.1)

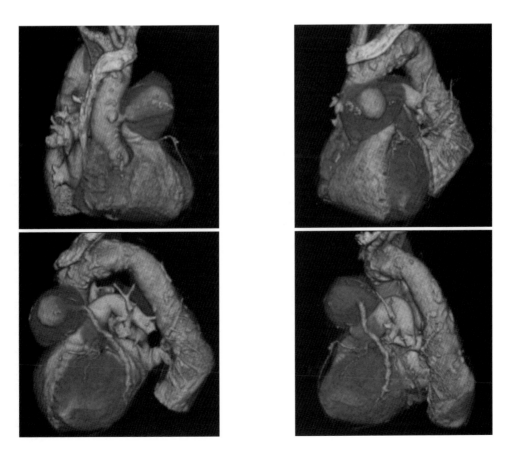

Figure 136 Bypass graft aneurysm (1.3)

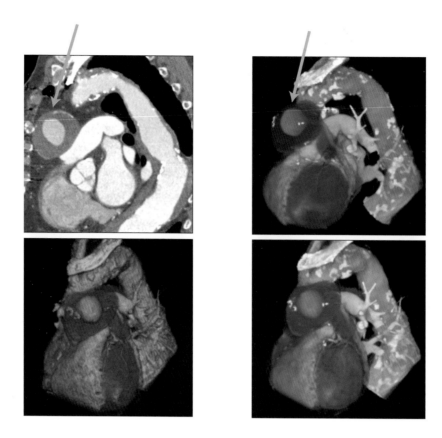

Figure 138 Bypass graft aneurysm (1.5)

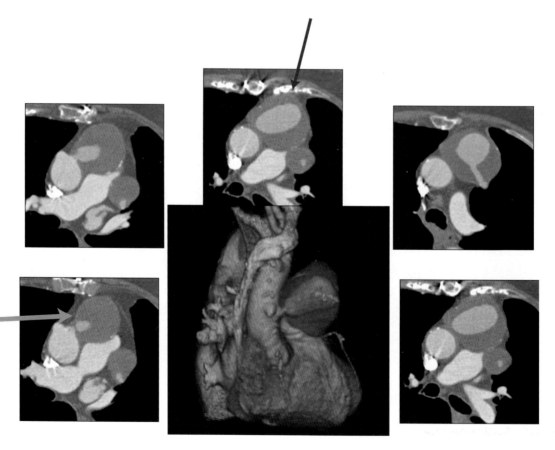

Figure 139 Bypass graft aneurysm (1.6)

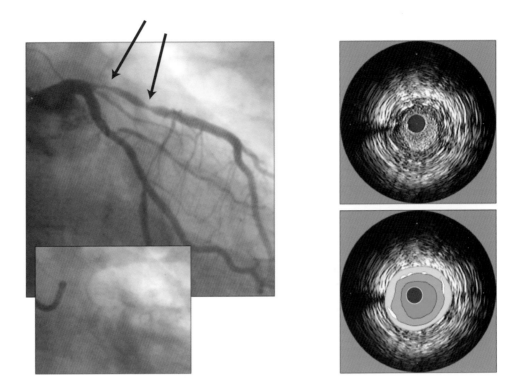

Figure 142   Coronary stent (1.1)

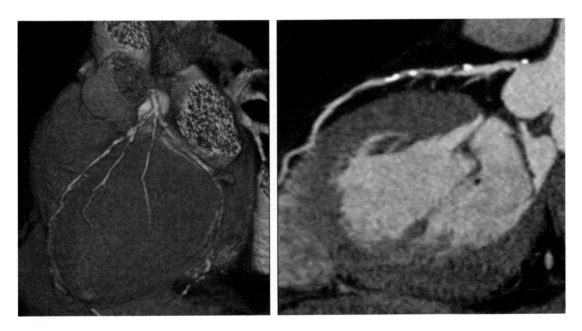

Figure 195   Aortic valve vegetation (1.2)

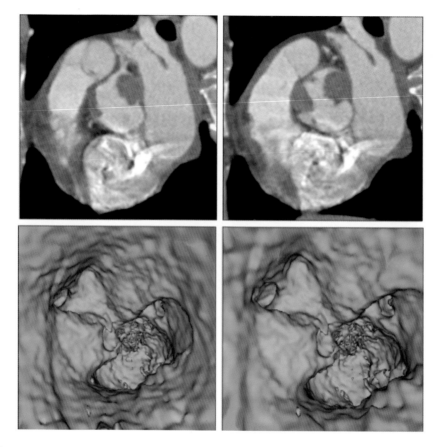

Figure 208 Aortic root mass (1.3)

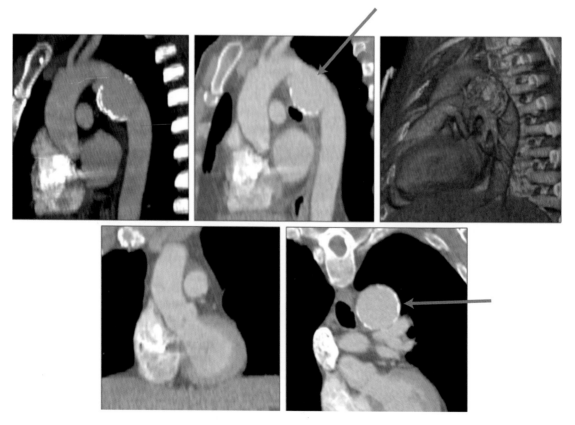

Figure 237 Post-traumatic aneurysm

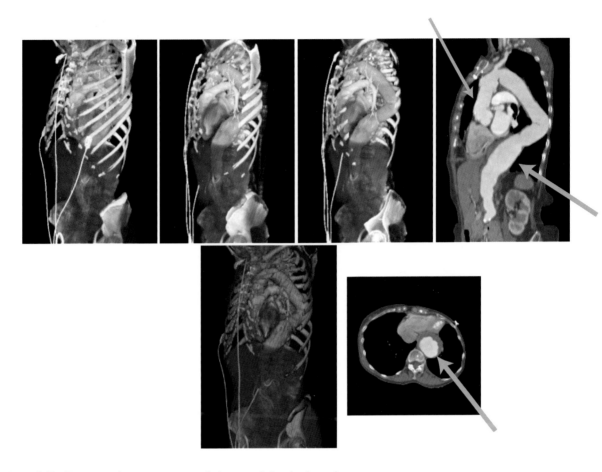

Figure 242   Preoperative assessment of thoracoabdominal aortic aneurysm

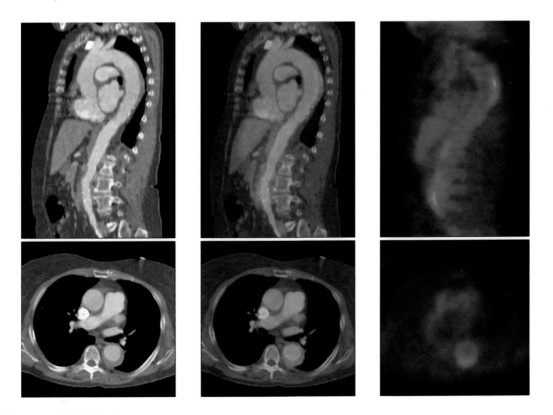

Figure 261   Aortitis PET/CT

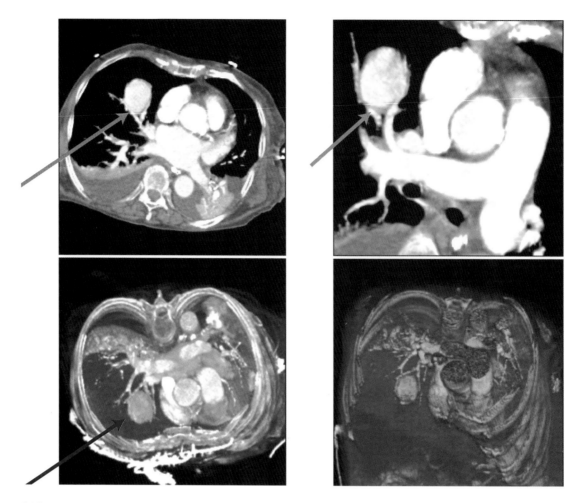

Figure 264   Pulmonary artery pseudoaneurysm

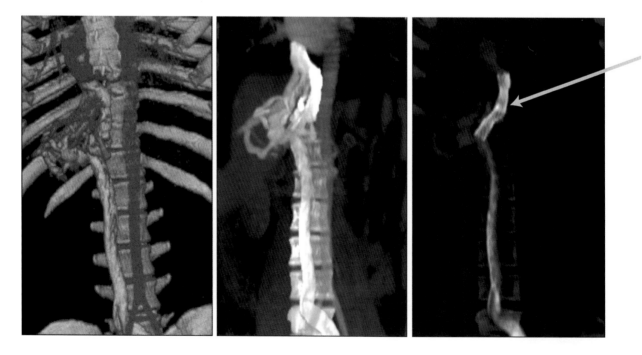

Figure 278   Stents in large collateral vessel of occluded inferior vena cava.

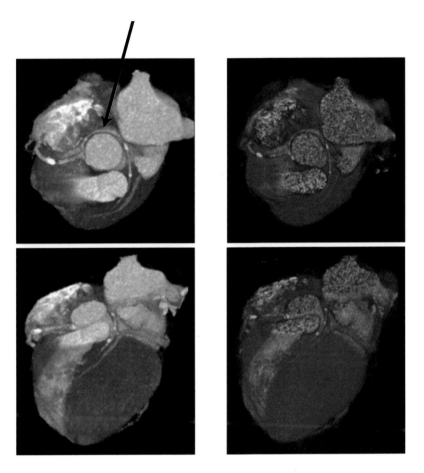

Figure 290   Anomalous coronary origin (5)

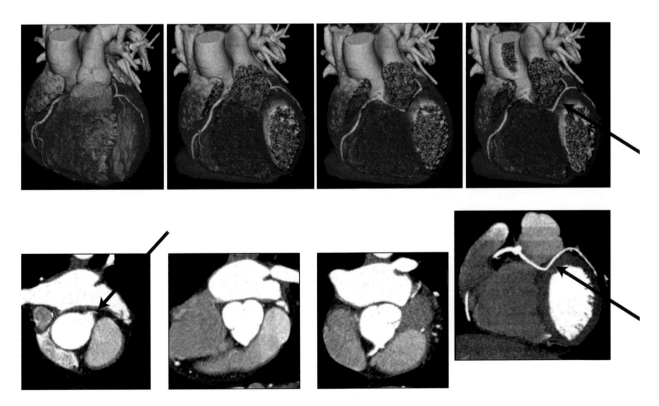

Figure 293   Anomalous coronary artery: intramyocardial course (7.2)

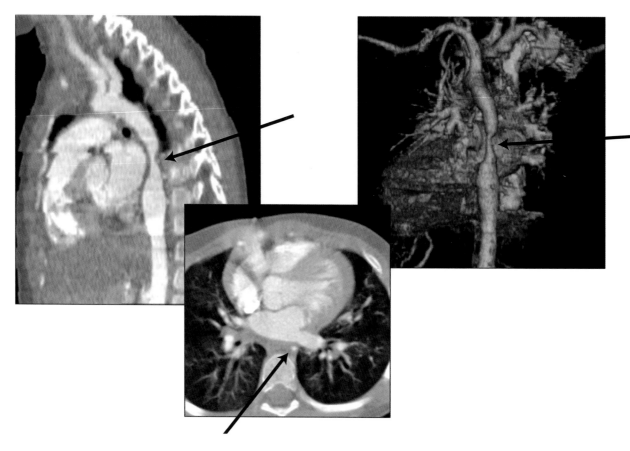

Figure 307   Coarctation of the aorta (2)

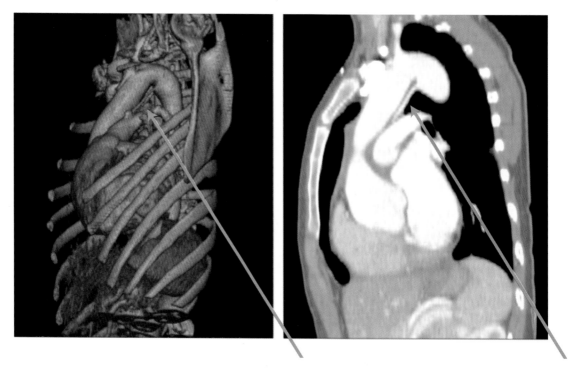

Figure 315   Patent ductus arteriosus (PDA)

1

Introduction

Over the past several years, computed tomography (CT) has assumed an important clinical role in the evaluation of cardiovascular disease. The clinical spectrum covers routine indications such as the assessment of aortic dissection as well as emerging applications including non-invasive assessment of the coronary anatomy.

Cardiovascular CT imaging is complementary to standard X-ray based imaging modalities and may allow novel diagnostic approaches, in particular the evaluation of early, asymptomatic stages of cardiovascular disease. *Planar* imaging modalities, including the chest X-ray and conventional angiographic techniques, project three-dimensional structures onto a two-dimensional image plane (Figure 1). The image reflects the X-ray attenuation of all the structures between X-ray tube and radiation detector, preventing the differentiation of individual structures. In contrast, the basic concept of CT is the reconstruction of a thin image slice from multiple projections obtained by rotating an X-ray source and detector system around the patient. In the resulting *tomographic* image, individual structures are differentiated by different image intensities (Figure 1)[1–3].

The advantages of tomographic CT imaging are partially offset by the lower temporal resolution or longer time required to obtain data for a single image (Figure 2). The temporal resolution is less relevant for imaging of large static organs (e.g. the kidney) and organs where motion can temporarily be suspended (e.g. lungs). However, because of the rapid, constant motion of the heart during the cardiac cycle, long acquisition times increase cardiac motion artifact (image blurring). The development of CT systems for cardiovascular imaging therefore required optimized acquisition times and synchro-

nization of imaging acquisition with the cardiac cycle.

1.1 IMPACT OF CT DEVELOPMENT ON CARDIOVASCULAR APPLICATIONS

Initial CT systems, introduced in 1972 for body imaging[3], rotated the X-ray tube and detector system very slowly around the patient. Because the power required to operate the X-ray tube was provided through attached cables, it was also necessary to return the gantry to its initial position after each slice acquisition. The patient table was then incremented to the next slice position, and scanning was repeated ('sequential' or 'step and shoot' scanning). Despite significant reduction of the rotation time to about 2 s by 1990, cardiovascular applications were still limited. Significant reduction of the acquisition time to allow synchronized imaging of a single view in a fraction of the RR interval (the time interval between two heartbeats, e.g. 1000 ms for a heart rate of 60 beats per minute (bpm)) was required for imaging of the heart, in order to reduce cardiac motion artifact (Figure 2) Further scanner development took two different directions: electron-beam CT (EBCT) and multidetector row CT (MDCT)[4].

EBCT scanners, which were specifically developed for cardiovascular imaging, generate the rotating X-ray beam by reflecting a rapidly undulating electron beam onto a stationary tungsten target ring encircling the patient (Figure 3). Eliminating the need to rotate the X-ray source mechanically around the patient, EBCT scanners significantly improved temporal resolution. Current

EBCT scanners can acquire one image slice in 30–100 ms. The acquisition of subsequent image slices occurs in consecutive cardiac cycles ('prospective triggering', see Chapter 2.1.3.1)[5,6].

Simultaneous with the development of EBCT, significant technical advances in mechanical CT systems, including spiral scanning and multidetector row technology, were realized. Changes in gantry design, with replacement of the connecting cables by slip rings, allowed transfer of the required electrical energy to a continuously rotating gantry, eliminating the previously required start–stop motion of the X-ray tube/detector system. Scanners with fast data acquisition during continuous rotation of the gantry and continuous movement of the patient table ('spiral' or 'helical' scanning) were introduced in 1989[7,8] (Figure 4). Reduction of gantry rotation time to less than 1 s per rotation and data acquisition synchronized to the electrocardiogram (ECG) signal with systems introduced in 1994 allowed cardiovascular imaging[9–13]. A second major advancement in mechanical CT systems was the introduction of scanners capable of acquiring more than one image per rotation. Scanners capable of fast simultaneous acquisition of two slices (dual-slice)[14–18] and four

slices[19,20] were introduced in 1994 and 1998, respectively. Four-slice scanners permitted ECG-synchronized data acquisition, rotation times as low as 500 ms, minimum slice thicknesses of 1.25 mm and maximum scan times for coverage of the entire heart equal to 35–40 s (Figure 5). Eight- and 16-slice scanners were introduced in 2001 and 2002, respectively[17, 21–25], and systems with acquisition of 40–64 slices per rotation in 2004. These scanners permit rotation times as low as 330 ms, minimum slice thickness of 0.75 mm and further reduced scan times.

As a result of these technical developments, clinical applications of cardiovascular CT have expanded. CT has already become a standard test for many clinical indications (e.g. imaging of the aorta, pulmonary embolism), and has great potential in the diagnosis of other common cardiovascular pathologies, including those of the coronary arteries. Currently, both EBCT and MDCT scanners are used for clinical cardiovascular imaging. This book is focused on cardiovascular multidetector CT imaging. Most of the images in the atlas are obtained with a 16-slice scanner, but the recent transition to 64-slice scanners is already reflected.

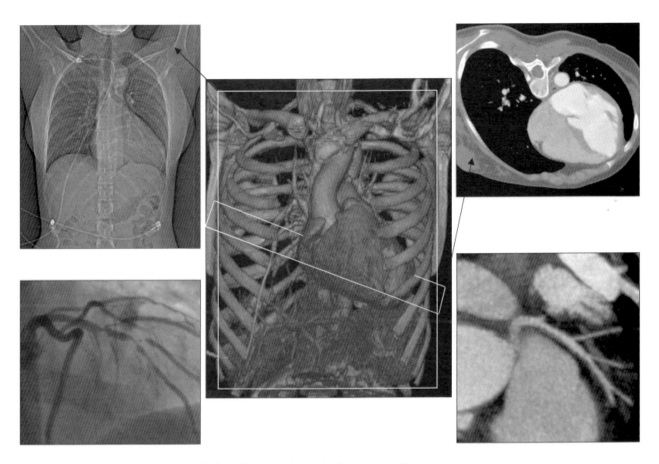

Figure 1 Planar versus tomographic imaging (see also color image on p.1)

Format: multiplanar reformation (MPR), volume-rendered image (VRI), planar X-ray, angiogram

Planar imaging modalities such as the chest X-ray and selective angiography project the three-dimensional structures onto a two-dimensional image plane. The image reflects the X-ray attenuation of all the structures between the X-ray tube and radiation detector, preventing the differentiation of individual structures. In contrast, the basic concept of computed tomography (CT) is the reconstruction of a thin image slice from multiple projections obtained by rotating an X-ray source and detector system around the patient. In the resulting tomographic image individual structures are differentiated by different image intensities.

The center panel of this figure shows a 3-D volume-rendered CT image of the chest. The panels on the left and right show planar and tomographic images, respectively. The standard chest X-ray (upper left panel) is a planar projection of the cardiac chambers. By filling the coronary arteries with contrast material, coronary angiography selectively enhances these structures (lower left panel). However, similar to the chest X-ray, the angiogram is a planar image, projecting the silhouette of the contrast-filled coronary artery lumen. The tomographic CT images of the cardiac chambers (right upper panel) and of a coronary artery (right lower panel) allow the visualization of details not seen with planar imaging.

CHAPTER 1, REFERENCES 1–3

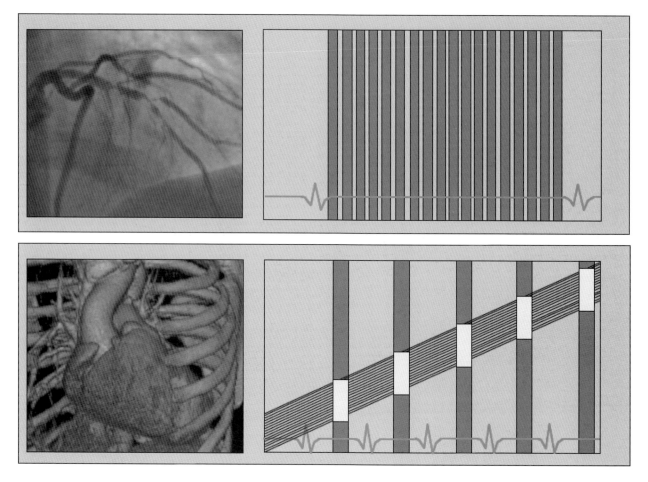

Figure 2   Image acquisition time (see also color image on p.1)

Format: VRI, angiogram, illustration

The advantages of tomographic CT imaging are partially offset by the lower temporal resolution or time required to obtain data for a single image. The temporal resolution is less critical for imaging of large static organs (e.g. the kidney) and organs where motion can temporarily be suspended (e.g. lungs). However, because of the rapid, constant motion of the heart during the cardiac cycle, cardiovascular CT presents significant technical challenges, which become obvious by a comparison with cine-angiography.

As demonstrated by the vertical bars in the upper part of the figure, cine-angiography acquires multiple image frames in one cardiac cycle. The time needed to acquire an individual planar image frame during cine-angiography is about 10 ms, allowing real-time imaging. In contrast, as shown in the lower part of the figure, the acquisition of an individual CT image slice is performed during late diastole of one cardiac cycle. The time required for the acquisition of an individual axial CT image with multidetector scanners is about 190 ms.

CHAPTER 1, REFERENCES 1–3

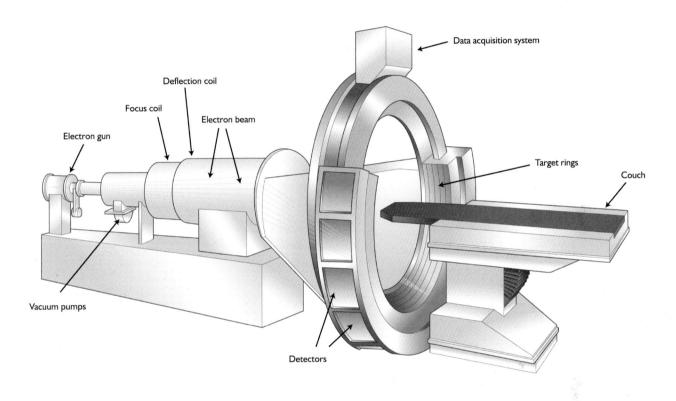

Figure 3   Electron beam CT technology (EBCT)

Format: illustration

EBCT scanners, which were specifically developed for cardiovascular imaging, generate a rotating X-ray beam by deflecting a rapidly undulating electron beam onto a stationary tungsten target ring encircling the patient. Eliminating the need to rotate the X-ray source mechanically around the patient, EBCT scanners significantly improve temporal resolution. Current EBCT scanners can acquire data for a single image slice in 30–100 ms.

CHAPTER 1.1, REFERENCES 4–6

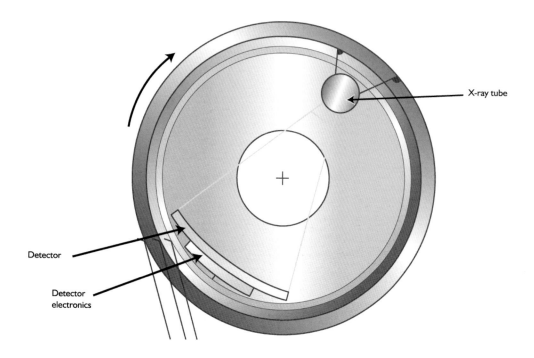

Figure 4   Spiral imaging with mechanical CT technology

Format: illustration

Simultaneous to the development of EBCT, significant technical advances of mechanical CT systems were realized. Changes in gantry design with replacement of the connecting cables by slip rings allowed transfer of the required electrical energy to a continuously rotating gantry, eliminating the previously required start–stop motion of the X-ray tube/detector system. Scanners with fast data acquisition during continuous rotation of the gantry and continuous movement of the patient table ('spiral' or 'helical' scanning) were introduced in 1989. Reduction of tube rotation time to less than 1 s per rotation and data acquisition synchronized to the electrocardiogram (ECG) signal with systems introduced in 1994 allowed cardiovascular imaging.

CHAPTER 1.1, REFERENCES 7–13

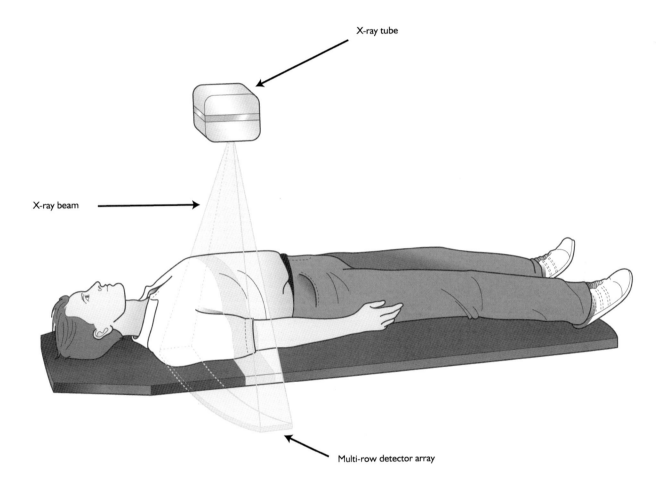

X-ray tube

X-ray beam

Multi-row detector array

Figure 5   Multidetector CT technology (MDCT)

Format: illustration

A second major advancement in mechanical CT systems was the introduction of scanners capable of acquiring more than one image per rotation. Scanners capable of simultaneous acquisition of two slices (dual-slice) and four- slices were introduced in 1994 and 1998, respectively. Four-slice scanners permitted ECG-synchronized data acquisition with rotation times as low as 500 ms, minimum slice thickness of 1.25 mm, and maximum scan times for coverage of the entire heart equal to 35–40 s. Eight- and 16-slice scanners were introduced in 2001 and 2002, respectively, and systems with acquisition of 40–64 slices per rotation are currently being introduced clinically. These scanners permit rotation times as low as 330 ms, minimum slice thickness of 0.75 mm and further reduced scan times.

CHAPTER 1.1, REFERENCES 14–25

2

Cardiovascular multidetector row computed tomography

2.1 TECHNICAL ASPECTS OF SCAN ACQUISITION

2.1.1 Current and future scanner systems

As described above, technical advances over the past several years have allowed the development of CT systems capable of cardiovascular imaging (Figure 6). However, significant limitations remain, which are related to the following requirements of cardiovascular imaging:

(1) High temporal resolution (fast image acquisition) to limit cardiac motion artifacts;

(2) High spatial resolution to visualize small cardiac anatomy;

(3) Isotropic voxels (identical spatial resolution in-plane and through-plane) to allow oblique reconstruction without loss of resolution;

(4) Fast volume coverage during one breath-hold period to reduce respiratory motion artifacts;

(5) ECG-synchronization of data acquisition.

The 16-slice systems used to obtain the majority of images in this atlas permit ECG-synchronized scanning with a gantry rotation time as fast as 375 ms and resulting temporal resolution of 190 ms. These systems achieve an in-plane spatial resolution of approximately 0.45 x 0.45 mm and a minimal slice thickness of 0.75 mm. The currently introduced generation of scanners with up to 64 slices and a gantry rotation time of 330 ms will come closer to the goal of imaging with isotropic voxels (Figures 7 and 8). The number of detector arrays also determines the volume covered in a single rotation.

For example, using a typical cardiac protocol with 0.75-mm slice thickness and a 16-slice scanner, one rotation covers a distance of 8 mm. Coverage of the entire heart in one rotation is currently not possible, and would require a significant increase in the number of detectors or flat-panel technology[26–28].

2.1.2 ECG referencing

The rapid, constant motion of the heart can cause significant image artifact. Cardiac motion varies throughout the cardiac cycle, with a peak and nadir in systole and diastole, respectively. It is therefore important to synchronize data acquisition to the cardiac cycle. Synchronization of data acquisition is also a prerequisite to combine data acquired from consecutive gantry rotations in volumetric datasets (Figure 9).

Typically, synchronization is based on observation of the ECG signal. The time between two consecutive heartbeats is described by the RR interval (the interval between consecutive R waves of the ECG, 1000 ms for a heart rate of 60 bpm). Depending on the acquisition mode, the RR interval of the ECG signal is used either prospectively to trigger data acquisition or retrospectively to gate data reconstruction to a certain phase of the cardiac cycle. The starting position of the data acquisition or reconstruction window is chosen in relation to the R wave of the ECG signal, typically using a relative delay value. The relative delay value is defined as a given percentage of the RR interval and automatically adapts to changing heart rates during the scan[29].

For morphologic evaluation, data are usually selected from the diastolic phase of the cardiac cycle where heart motion is minimal, using either a relative delay of 40–60% or an absolute delay of 300–500 ms before the next R wave. However, the precise phase with minimal motion is patient-, scanner- and heart rate-dependent and should be optimized to ensure maximum image quality (Figure 10)[30,31]. In addition, several reconstructions may be necessary, because different structures may reach minimal motion in slightly different phases of the cardiac cycle (e.g. left versus right coronary artery). Importantly, data can also be chosen from multiple phases throughout the cardiac cycle for functional evaluation (Figures 11 and 12) (Movies 1 and 2).

2.1.3 Acquisition mode

2.1.3.1 Sequential (axial) mode

Early mechanical CT systems required the gantry to return to its initial position after each image slice acquisition. Individual transaxial image slices were acquired, followed by incremental advancement of the patient table and repeated image acquisition at the next level (the 'step and shoot' mode). Modern multidetector row computed tomography (MDCT) scanners can be operated in this sequential mode, which is still used for some applications (e.g. calcium scoring). Data acquisition is prospectively triggered by the ECG signal, typically in late diastole (prospective triggering). An advantage of the sequential mode is lower radiation dose, because X-ray exposure only occurs during the prospectively triggered cardiac phase rather than throughout the entire cardiac cycle. Limitations of sequential acquisition include the increased sensitivity to motion artifact, because prospective referencing of the ECG signal restricts image reconstruction to a single phase of the cardiac cycle. In addition, examination times are increased because of the need to increment the patient table between slice acquisitions.

2.1.3.2 Spiral (helical) mode

As described in Chapter 1.1, the development of multidetector row scanners together with spiral acquisition technology has been crucial for cardiovascular imaging. Consequently, advanced cardiovascular MDCT imaging is predominantly performed in the spiral mode. In the spiral mode, data are acquired during constant rotation of the X-ray tube/detector system and continuous movement of the patient table through the gantry. This type of data acquisition results in true three-dimensional volumetric series. Data are acquired throughout the entire cardiac cycle with simultaneous recording of the ECG signal. Data from specific periods of the cardiac cycle (most commonly late diastole) are then used for image reconstruction by retrospective referencing to the ECG signal (retrospective ECG gating)[32,33] (Figure 9). Importantly, because data are acquired throughout the cardiac cycle, spiral imaging allows reconstruction during multiple cardiac phases, which is important for coronary imaging (Figure 10) and required for functional assessment (Figures 11 and 12) (Movies 1 and 2). Spiral, retrospectively ECG-gated techniques are less sensitive to arrhythmia, and allow faster volume coverage with improved through-plane resolution. Because image acquisition and therefore X-ray exposure occurs throughout the cardiac cycle, the improved image quality with spiral techniques is generally associated with higher patient radiation doses compared with imaging using traditional sequential techniques.

2.1.4 Special image reconstruction to improve temporal resolution

Modern CT scanners use special imaging reconstruction techniques to improve temporal resolution. These include partial scan reconstructions and segmented reconstructions.

2.1.4.1 Partial scan reconstruction

Partial scan reconstruction algorithms reconstruct the individual axial image from data obtained during less than one complete rotation of the X-ray tube[4,34] Because only 180° of the projection data are needed for reconstruction, the temporal resolution for each axial image is reduced to one-half of the gantry rotation time. These protocols are used with sequential and spiral image acquisitions and are the norm for cardiovascular CT systems.

2.1.4.2 Segmented reconstruction

Used with spiral data acquisition, segmented reconstruction algorithms can further improve temporal resolution[35–38] Segmented algorithms obtain the data required for reconstruction of an individual image from several consecutive cardiac cycles. Therefore, the duration of the acquisition window in each cycle can be reduced. These algorithms are particularly useful for patients with elevated heart rates, which are associated with significantly shorter diastolic windows of minimal motion. However, the improvement in temporal resolution achieved with segmented reconstruction algorithms depends on the relationship between the gantry rotation time and the patient's heart rate, and optimal temporal resolution is only achieved for certain combinations of heart rate and gantry rotation time. Therefore, prospective selection of gantry rotation from multiple discrete values based on patient heart rates prior to scanning has been proposed. However, because the heart rate typically varies slightly during the examination, consistent achievement of the optimal temporal resolution would require dynamic adjustment of the gantry rotation speed. The number of heart cycles used for segmented reconstruction of spiral data is limited by several factors, and a maximum of two segments is usually recommended for morphologic imaging. Therefore, segmented reconstructions typically result in temporal resolutions as low as 84–165 ms with the newest scanners.

2.1.5 Radiation exposure and tube current modulation

2.1.5.1 Radiation exposure

The radiation exposure during a CT examination depends on the image protocol, which is dictated by the clinical question. The effective patient radiation dose is small for calcium scoring, but comparable to that of conventional selective coronary angiography during MDCT coronary angiography[39–42].

2.1.5.2 Tube current modulation

The higher patient radiation dose with spiral compared with sequential techniques is in part the result of continuous X-ray exposure during the entire cardiac cycle. However, for most current clinical indications, only data from the diastolic phase are typically used for image reconstruction. Some modern scanners therefore allow reduction of the tube current outside the selected (diastolic) phase to decrease patient radiation exposure[43] (Figure 13). Therefore, tube current and image quality are at a maximum only during the selected cardiac phase, but are reduced by about 80% outside this phase.

From a clinical point of view, it is important to consider that although data are available during the entire cardiac cycle, image quality outside the selected (diastolic) phase is limited. Therefore, reconstruction at different phases, e.g. for coronary imaging (Figure 10) or functional imaging (Figures 11 and 12), is limited.

2.1.6 Contrast media

Most cardiovascular protocols require the intravenous administration of iodinated contrast agents to enhance selective cardiovascular structures. Patients with renal insufficiency or contrast allergy are either pretreated (e.g. hydration, steroid treatment) or imaged with alternative modalities. Standard contrast agents with an iodine concentration of 300–400 mg/ml are injected into an antecubital vein using power injectors with injection rates of 2.5–4 ml/s. If peripheral access is not available, hand injection in a central vein can be considered. The amount of contrast agent required for a cardiac scan varies between 100 and 150 ml, depending on the scan protocol and the scanner type.

Currently available contrast media are quickly diluted in the blood and distributed into the extracellular space, providing only a short time window for enhanced imaging. The transit time from the standard injection site (antecubital vein) to the heart is patient dependent, and can vary between 20 and 40 s. Therefore, determination of scan delay (time between the start of contrast agent injection and the start of the scan) is critical to ensure optimal enhancement of the desired cardiovascular structures[44]. This can be achieved with a small 'timing bolus' or by monitoring the diagnostic bolus ('bolus tracking'). With the use of a timing bolus, approximately 20 ml of contrast agent are injected and an individual slice (typically at a level ~ 2 cm below the carina for imaging of the aorta) is repeatedly imaged (Figure 14). Based on the resulting enhancement curve of the descending aorta, transit time to the region of interest (ROI) is determined and used for timing of the diagnostic bolus. Alternatively, with bolus monitoring techniques, the entire diagnostic bolus is injected, and contrast enhancement is monitored in the ROI by repeated imaging at a single level. Once a certain enhancement threshold is achieved, breath-hold instructions are given and scanning is started.

Bolus injection of contrast can lead to inhomogeneous enhancement, in particular in the superior vena cava (SVC) and right atrium (RA), where enhanced and non-enhanced blood meet (Figure 15) (see Chapter 2.2.5.5). Non-uniform enhancement and the resulting beam-hardening artifacts may obscure right-sided structures such as the pulmonary vessels and right coronary artery. Ongoing research evaluates the impact of different injection protocols and contrast agents. Artifacts in the SVC and RA may be reduced by scanning in the caudal–cranial direction and by the injection of a saline bolus following the contrast agent[45–47]. Similarly, contrast injection at variable flow rates has been proposed to provide more prolonged, uniform enhancement of the aorta[48,49].

In patients with iodine contrast allergy or renal insufficiency, CT scanning with gadolinium-based magnetic resonance imaging (MRI) contrast materials can provide an alternative (Figure 16).

2.1.7 Control of heart rate: beta-blocker

Because of the association of lower heart rates with longer diastolic windows of minimal cardiac motion, cardiovascular CT image quality is improved for stable, slow heart rates (optimally around 60 bpm). This is particularly important if small structures, including the coronary arteries, are examined. Although modern scanners allow correction for arrhythmia and higher heart rates ('segmented reconstruction', Chapter 2.1.4.2), heart rate control with an intravenous or oral beta-blocker is preferred by many groups, if no contraindications exist (e.g. significant asthma, heart failure, aortic stenosis, heart block)[50,51] (see Appendix 6.2).

2.1.8 Control of vessel tone: nitroglycerin

In analogy to conventional cardiac catheterization, CT coronary angiography (CTA) is often performed after sublingual administration of small nitroglycerin doses. The rationale is that visualization of a dilated vessel is improved (see Appendix 6.3).

2.1.9 Imaging protocols

A critical step in obtaining clinically meaningful results is careful planning of the CT examination protocol according to the specific clinical indication. High-resolution, retrospective ECG-gated techniques with minimal slice thickness are usually reserved for visualization of small cardiac anatomy (e.g. coronary arteries). Imaging of the aorta is performed with retrospective ECG-gated techniques with larger slice thickness. Lower-resolution, lower-dose sequential or spiral techniques are used for calcium screening.

2.2 IMAGE RECONSTRUCTION AND INTERPRETATION

The acquisition of images with MDCT is performed in the axial plane (Figure 17). Review of the axial images allows the experienced reader to gain an understanding of the overall anatomy. However, since the axes of the heart and the vascular structures are oblique to the axial plane, additional data manipulation with reconstruction of the volumetric data set into oblique planes is almost always performed (Figures 18 and 19). The image processing techniques most often used are two-dimensional (2-D) multiplanar reformation (MPR) and maximum intensity projection (MIP), 3-D shaded surface display (SSD) and volume rendering (VR) and 4-D volume rendering[52]. The quality of these reformatted images depends on the in-plane and through-plane spatial resolution. If the through-plane resolution or slice thickness is larger than the in-plane resolution of axial images, oblique reformation will be associated with a loss of spatial resolution compared with the axial images. It is anticipated that future systems with isotopic voxels will allow oblique reformation without loss of resolution. It is also important to understand that advanced 3-D and 4-D displays of the CT data can be associated with loss of image detail. Experienced CT readers, therefore, always confirm findings on the axial 'source' images.

2.2.1 The axial CT image

Because current CT systems still have higher in-plane than through-plane resolution, the axial 'source' images have the highest spatial resolution (Figure 17). Therefore, the initial step for the interpretation of CT images remains review of the individual tomographic transaxial image slices, and findings on reconstructed images should always be confirmed in the axial images.

2.2.2 Two-dimensional reformation

The strength of volumetric 3-D CT imaging is that image processing allows reformation in unlimited planes not specified at the time of data acquisition. This is critically important for cardiac imaging, because most cardiac axes are oblique to the axial plane. Interactive computer workstations allow the user to place orthogonal planes through the data set, creating sagittal and frontal images. Further manipulation of the reformatted plane provides oblique images, following the orientation of cardiac structures, for example the left ventricle or the aorta (Figures 20 and 21). In addition, curved planes that follow the course of, for example, tortuous vessels can be created by tracing the path of the vessel on the original axial images (Figures 22 and 23). The resulting curved image displays the 3-D course of the vessel. However, the surrounding anatomy is sometimes distorted in these images.

The axial 'source' image is a 2-D gray-scale image displaying all pixels in an individual image slice with the thickness chosen for image acquisition. 2-D images can be reconstructed in different formats at an arbitrary slice thickness. The simplest reconstruction method for visualization is the multiplanar reformation (MPR) (Figure 24). An MPR is a 2-D image displaying all pixels in a chosen plane. The original CT values are preserved. Therefore, in a contrast-enhanced MPR image of, for example, a coronary vessel, both the high-intensity signal of the contrast-filled lumen and the low-intensity signal of the vessel wall are represented. Another common reconstruction technique is the maximum intensity projection (MIP). In contrast to the MPR, the MIP is a 2-D image displaying only the maximum intensity pixels (Figure 24). Therefore, in a contrast-enhanced MIP image of the coronary vessel, visualization of the lumen is optimized but the wall structures are less well seen. Because of their similarity to conventional angiographic images, MIP images are often used for CT angiography. However, only part of the original CT data are preserved, and findings should be confirmed on MPR images.

2.2.3 Three-dimensional reformation

Volume-rendered reconstruction employs advanced 3-D image processing algorithms with semi-transparent visualization of superficial and deep contours. Each voxel is assigned a value for opacity according to its CT number, such that lower-intensity tissues are more transparent whereas higher-intensity tissues are more opaque. Therefore, the more opaque tissue is visible through translucent tissue, creating depth perception. Volume-rendered (VR) images allow demonstration of complex anatomy and appreciation of the spatial relationship between visualized structures (Figure 25) (Movie 3). Levels of opacity can be varied to alter the display of data as needed. In addition, the VR data can be viewed at arbitrary angles, including the standard

views of conventional coronary angiography[53]. Color coding can also be used to further enhance the 3-D appearance (Figure 26).

Perspective volume rendering (pVR) provides virtual endoscopic views of the surface of anatomic structures that are sufficiently contrasted from surrounding tissue[54]. This technique is used to visualize cavities or tubular structures accessible to endoscopes (e.g. the colon or the bronchial tree). Although the clinical value is unclear, pVR can also be applied to chambers of the heart or vascular structures, which can be viewed from within by rendering blood transparent[55] (Figure 27). Tubular structures such as the coronary arteries can be viewed with motion along a path simulating flight through the vessel (Movie 4).

2.2.4 Four-dimensional reconstruction: dynamic imaging

Using retrospective ECG-gated spiral techniques, modern CT technology allows reconstruction of data for functional assessment (e.g. ejection fraction calculation). Multiple image sets from different phases in the cardiac cycle are reconstructed and combined into a cine-loop to produce a dynamic image set[56] (Figure 11) (Movies 1 and 2). These images allow qualitative assessment of, for example, left ventricular function and dynamic visualization of the complete spatial 3-D data set (true 4-D imaging) (Movie 5). However, the emerging results of dynamic CT imaging need to be further validated against established functional imaging modalities, in particular echocardiography and MRI[57].

2.2.5 Image artifacts

The recognition of image artifacts is important in order to avoid false-positive diagnosis. Artifacts are often related to patient characteristics and technical limitations of CT[58].

2.2.5.1 Cardiac motion artifact

Because of the rapid motion of the heart and the relatively long acquisition window, blurring of the image occurs, in particular if the acquisition window is not synchronized to the cardiac cycle (Chapter 2.1.2). An important example is motion artifact at the root of the aorta in non-gated studies (Figure 28). This artifact becomes more significant if smaller structures including the coronary arteries are imaged.

2.2.5.2 Arrhythmia Artifact

A typical motion artifact can be seen in patients with arrhythmia, particularly atrial fibrillation. As shown in Figures 29 and 30, typical band-like shifts of the image data are seen in image reconstructions. Each band represents the data obtained during one tube rotation and one heartbeat. Because of the irregular heart rate, data acquisition occurs at slightly different phases in subsequent cardiac cycles. Changes in ventricular size during systole and diastole can, therefore, lead to misregistration of images. Similar artifacts occur in patients with extrasystolic beats (Figures 31 and 32). Some modern CT systems allow editing of the detected R peaks of the ECG signal and improvements of cardiac motion artifact.

2.2.5.3 Partial volume averaging: blooming artifact

Small structures with high CT numbers, for example calcium or metallic material (coronary stents, surgical clips), cause a characteristic artifact, which often precludes assessment of adjacent structures[59,60]. This 'partial volume averaging' or 'blooming' artifact is related to the fact that an object with a high CT number, which is smaller than the voxel size, will increase the CT number of the overall voxel, represented on the CT image. Therefore, the object size is overestimated ('blooming') (Figures 8, 26 and 33–35).

2.2.5.4 Streak artifact: metallic implants

Large areas of high-density material, in particular metallic foreign bodies, can severely reduce X-ray transmission. In the extreme, the detector may not record any signal transmission, causing the reconstruction algorithm to fail, and produce streaks in the image originating from the source object. This has implications for cardiovascular imaging as metal implants are common. Examples are pacer/implantable cardioverter defibrillator wires, endovascular stents and surgical material (Figure 34).

2.2.5.5 Streak artifact: contrast material

Similar streak artifact is also caused by the contrast bolus injection. Particularly in the superior vena cava and right atrium, high-iodine-concentration contrast material and areas of mixing between contrast-rich and unenhanced blood can cause significant artifact, often precluding assessment of adjacent structures (Chapter 2.1.6) (Figure 15).

2.2.5.6 Noise

In patients with arrhythmia, images reconstructed from data acquired using dose-modulation techniques (Chapter 2.1.5) can lead to characteristic differences in signal-to-noise ratio in consecutive axial image slices, causing bands of different image quality in oblique images (Figure 13).

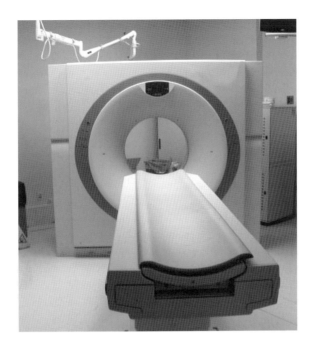

Figure 6   MDCT scanner

Format: photograph

Technical advances over the past several years have allowed the development of CT systems capable of cardiovascular imaging. 16-detector systems enable fast scanning (375 ms/rotation with 190 ms temporal resolution) of thin image slices (0.75 mm) with high in-plane spatial resolution of approximately 0.45 × 0.45 mm. Scanners able to acquire up to 64 slices in one rotation with faster gantry rotation are currently becoming available.

CHAPTER 2.1.1, REFERENCES 14–25

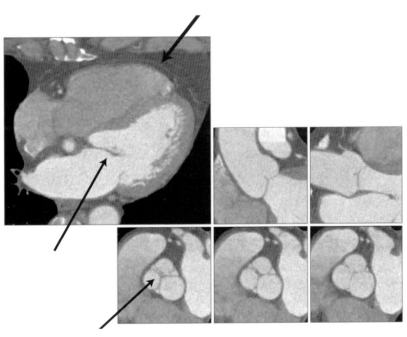

Figure 7   64-slice MDCT technology (1)

Format: MPR (64-slice)

This figure shows images obtained with a 64-slice MDCT system. The high resolution is reflected in the detailed visualization of the mitral and aortic valve leaflets (thin arrows) and the pericardium (thick arrow).

CHAPTER 2.1.1, REFERENCES 25–27

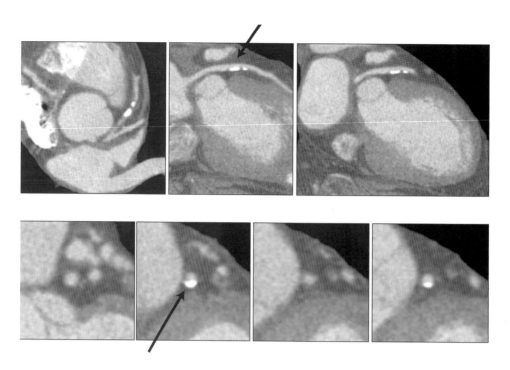

Figure 8   64-slice MDCT technology (2)

Format: MPR (64-slice)

This figure shows longitudinal and cross-sectional images of a left anterior descending (LAD) coronary artery obtained with a 64-slice system. The high resolution is demonstrated by the decreased blooming artifact (arrows) of the calcified plaque in the mid-LAD segment, allowing differentiation between lumen and plaque.

CHAPTER 2.1.1, REFERENCES 25–27

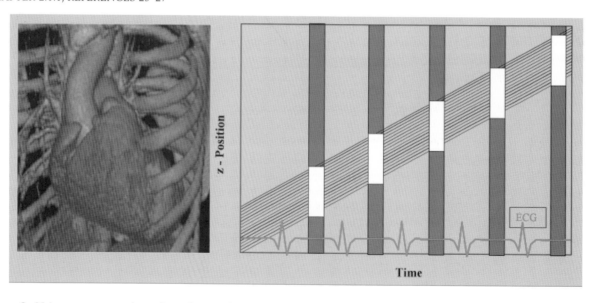

Figure 9   Volume coverage (see also color section on p. 2)

Format: VRI, illustration

The volume covered in a single rotation is determined by the number of detectors and slice thickness. For example, using a protocol with 0.75 mm slice thickness and a 16-slice scanner, one rotation covers a distance of 8 mm. Therefore, with current systems, coverage of the entire heart (10–20 cm) requires combining data acquired from subsequent tube rotations in subsequent heartbeats into the three-dimensional data set. Coverage of the entire heart in one rotation is currently not possible and would require a significant increase in the number of detectors or cone-beam technology.

CHAPTER 2.1.2, REFERENCES 29

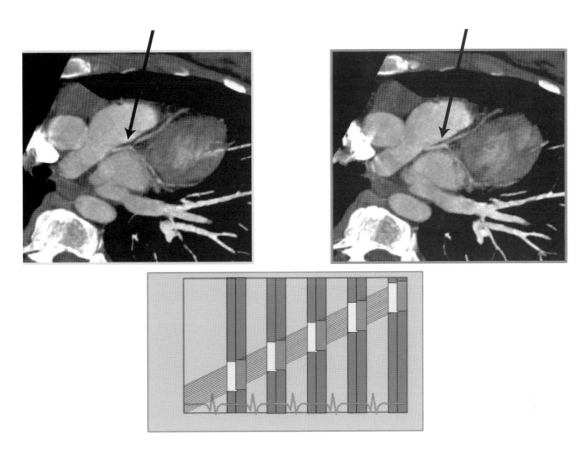

Figure 10 Reconstruction window: image quality (see also color section on p. 2)

Format: MPR, illustration

For morphologic evaluation, data are usually selected from the diastolic phase of the cardiac cycle where heart motion is minimal, using either a relative delay of 40–60% or an absolute delay of 300–500 ms before the next R wave. However, the precise phase with minimal motion is patient- and heart rate-dependent and should be optimized to ensure maximum image quality. In addition, reconstruction at several phases may be necessary, because different structures may reach minimal motion in slightly different phases of the cardiac cycle (e.g. left versus right coronary artery).

In this figure, the left anterior descending coronary artery of a young patient with atypical chest pain is shown. The data set was reconstructed at two different phases of the cardiac cycle. The apparent stenosis at the ostium of the LAD (arrow) is not confirmed on the additional data reconstruction, performed at a later phase.

CHAPTER 2.1.2, REFERENCES 30, 31

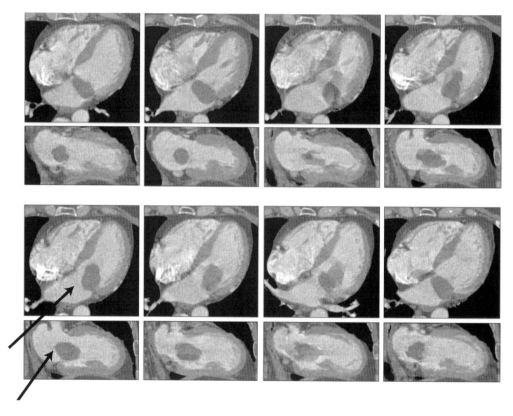

Figure 11   Functional assessment (1)

Format: MPR

For morphologic evaluation, data are usually selected from the diastolic phase of the cardiac cycle, where heart motion is minimal and image quality optimal. Importantly, data can also be reconstructed from multiple phases throughout the cardiac cycle for functional evaluation. Multiple image sets are then combined into a cine-loop to produce a dynamic image set (Movies 1 and 2).

This approach is exemplified in this figure, showing a mass (arrows) which is attached to the posterior aspect of the mitral annulus. Its mobility is demonstrated in consecutive phases of the cardiac cycle, during which the mass passes through the mitral valve plane.

CHAPTER 2.1.2, 2.2.4, REFERENCES 56, 57

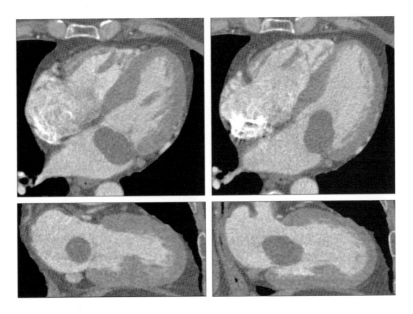

Figure 12   Functional assessment (2)

Format: MPR

Systolic and diastolic frames from the previous figure are shown in the left and right panels, respectively. The mass (probably a myxoma) is attached to the posterior aspect of the mitral annulus. During diastole it passes through the mitral valve plane.

CHAPTER 2.1.2, 2.2.4, REFERENCES 56, 57

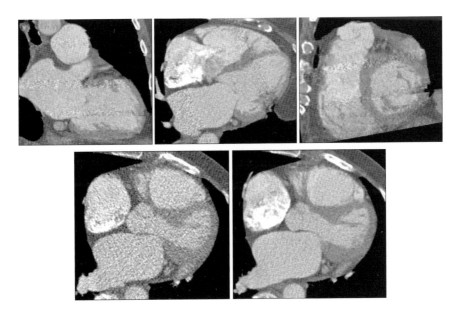

Figure 13   Dose modulation

Format: MPR

The higher patient radiation dose with spiral compared with sequential techniques is in part the result of continuous X-ray exposure during the entire cardiac cycle. However, for most current clinical indications typically only data from the diastolic phase are used for image reconstruction. Modern scanners therefore allow reduction of the tube current outside the selected (diastolic) phase to decrease patient radiation exposure. Therefore, tube current and image quality are maximal only during the selected cardiac phase, but are reduced by about 80% outside this phase.

This is demonstrated in the images of the heart from a patient in atrial fibrillation scanned with dose modulation. The oblique images in the upper row demonstrate bands of lower resolution, representing data acquisition outside the phase of maximum tube current. The difference in resolution in axial images is demonstrated in the lower part of the figure.

CHAPTER 2.1.5.2, REFERENCES 43

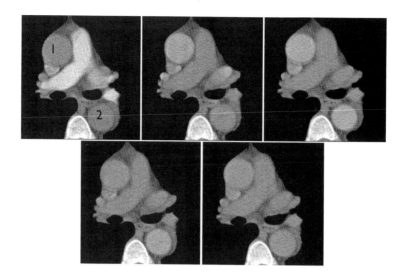

Figure 14   Test bolus

Format: MPR

Determination of scan delay (time between the start of contrast agent injection and the start of the scan) is critical to ensure optimal enhancement of the desired cardiovascular structures. This can be achieved with a small 'timing bolus' or 'bolus tracking'. With the use of a timing bolus, approximately 20 ml of contrast agent are injected and an individual image slice (typically at a level ~ 2 cm below the carina for imaging of the aorta) is repeatedly imaged. Based on the resulting enhancement curve of the ascending aorta, transit time is determined.

In this figure enhancement of the ascending (1) and the descending (2) aorta during the injection of a contrast bolus is shown. The left upper panel shows enhancement of the pulmonary artery, the right upper panel shows greater enhancement of the ascending than the descending aorta and the lower left panel greater enhancement of the descending than the ascending aorta.

CHAPTER 2.1.6, REFERENCES 44

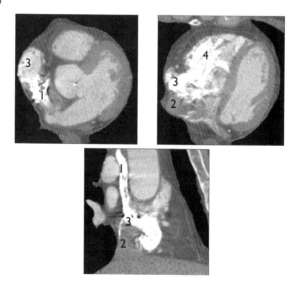

Figure 15 Streak artifact: contrast material

Format: MPR

Bolus injection of contrast leads to inhomogeneous enhancement, in particular of the superior vena cava (SVC) and right atrium (RA), where enhanced and non-enhanced blood mix. Non-uniform enhancement and the resulting beam-hardening artifacts may obscure right-sided structures such as the pulmonary vessels and right coronary artery.

This figure shows axial images at the interface between the SVC (1) and RA (3) (left upper) and inferior vena cava (IVC) (2) and RA (right upper) and a sagittal reconstruction (lower panel). Streak artifact is seen in the SVC, RA and right ventricle (RV) (4).

CHAPTER 2.1.6, 2.2.5.5, REFERENCES 45–47

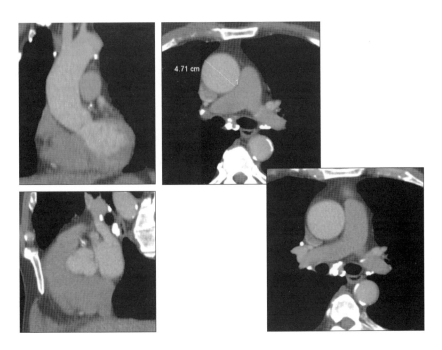

Figure 16   Gadolinium-enhanced CT

Format: MPR

In patients with iodine-contrast allergy or renal insufficiency, CT scanning with gadolinium-based magnetic resonance imaging (MRI) contrast materials can provide an alternative. Despite the decreased enhancement of the lumen, modified protocols are often diagnostic, in particular when used for aortic imaging. This is shown in this figure for a patient with mild prominence of the mid-ascending aorta.

CHAPTER 2.1.6 REFERENCES

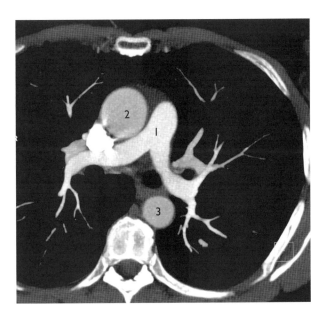

Figure 17   Axial image

Format: MPR

The acquisition of images with MDCT is performed in the axial plane. The review of these axial 'source' images allows the experienced reader to gain an understanding of the overall anatomy. Findings on reconstructed images should always be confirmed in the axial images.

In this figure, an example of an individual axial image at the level of the pulmonary artery bifurcation (1) is shown. The ascending (2) and the descending (3) aorta are seen.

CHAPTER 2.2, 2.2.1, REFERENCES 52

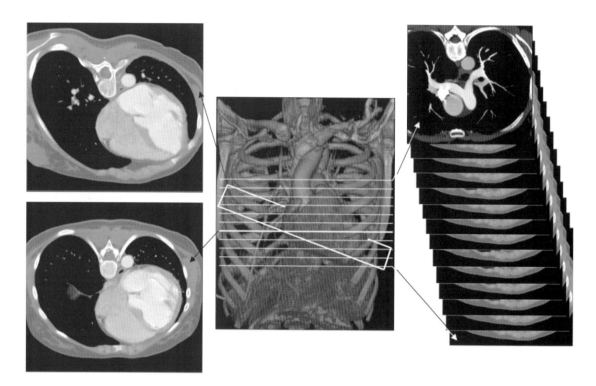

Figure 18   Axial and oblique images (see also color section on p. 3)

Format: VRI, MPR

The acquisition of images with MDCT is performed to the axial plane. Review of the tomographic, transaxial image stack (right side of the figure) allows the experienced reader to gain an understanding of the overall anatomy. However, since the axes of the heart and the vascular structures are oblique to the axial images, additional data manipulation with reconstruction of the volumetric datasets into oblique planes is almost always necessary.

This is demonstrated by the two images on the left. The near four-chamber view in the axial image (left lower panel) demonstrates foreshortening, particularly of the apex. The true four-chamber view oblique to the axial image demonstrates the true left ventricular geometry (left upper panel).

CHAPTER 2.2, 2.2.2, REFERENCE 52

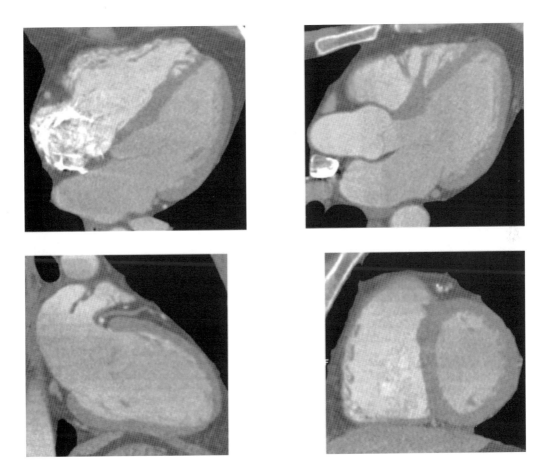

Figure 19   Imaging in oblique planes

Format: MPR

The strength of volumetric 3-D CT imaging is that image processing using computer workstations allows subsequent reformation in unlimited planes not specified at the time of data acquisition. Oblique reconstructions are performed using advanced 2-D, 3-D and 4-D rendering techniques.

In this figure typical oblique planes for the reconstruction of ventricular anatomy are demonstrated, including four-chamber (left upper), three-chamber (right upper), two-chamber (left lower) and short-axis (right lower) views.

CHAPTER 2.2, 2.2.2, REFERENCES 52

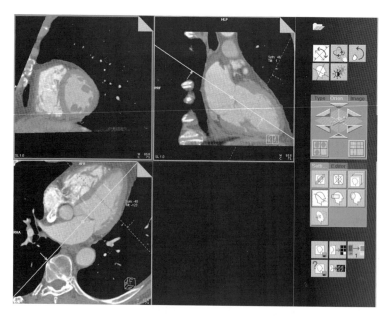

Figure 20   3-D workstation (1): oblique planes, left ventricle (see also color section on p. 3)

Format: MPR

Interactive computer workstations allow on-line analysis of the 3-D data set. Reconstruction of the volumetric datasets into oblique planes is performed, often matching planes used in other imaging modalities (e.g. echocardiography and magnetic resonance imaging).

This image demonstrates the reconstruction of a short-axis view of the left ventricle (left upper panel). Adjusting the image plane (interrupted line in upper right and lower left images) perpendicular to the left ventricular axis provides a true short-axis view.

CHAPTER 2.2.2, REFERENCES 52

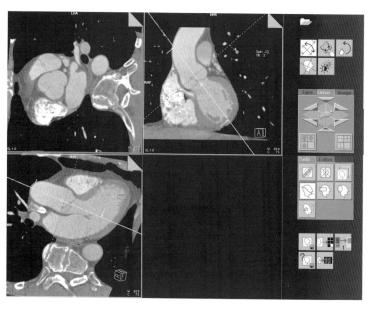

Figure 21   3-D workstation (2): oblique planes, aortic root (see also color section on p. 4)

Format: MPR

Another example of reconstruction of a typically used image plane is shown in this figure. It demonstrates the reconstruction of the aortic root, showing the sinuses of Valsalva and valve leaflets (left upper panel). Adjusting the image plane (interrupted line in upper right and lower left images) perpendicular to the ascending aorta provides a true perpendicular cut through the aortic root.

CHAPTER 2.2.2, REFERENCES 52

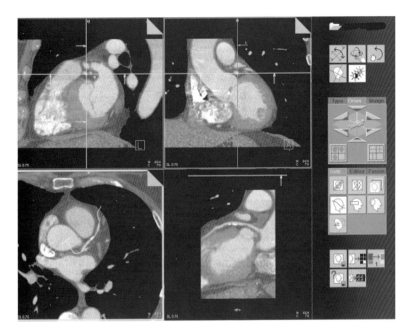

Figure 22 Curved 2-D reconstruction (1) (see also color section on p. 4)

Format: MPR

In addition to oblique planes, curved planes that follow the course of, for example, tortuous vessels can be created by tracing the path of the vessel on the original axial images. The resulting curved image displays the 3-D course of the vessel and surrounding anatomy.

In this figure a curved MPR of the proximal and mid-LAD is shown (right lower panel). The left lower panel demonstrates the reconstructed course of the LAD through the axial images.

CHAPTER 2.2.2, REFERENCES 52

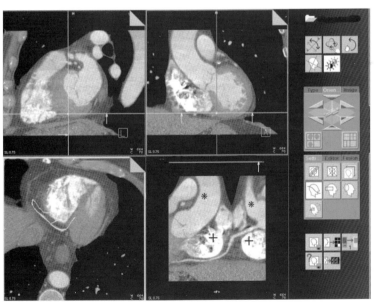

Figure 23 Curved 2-D reconstruction (2) (see also color section on p. 5)

Format: MPR (64-slice)

This figure demonstrates that in these curved MPR images the anatomy of the cardiovascular structures surrounding the displayed vessel is sometimes distorted.

In this curved MPR of the right coronary artery (RCA), the ascending aorta (*) and right atrium (+) are visible in a 'mirror' image.

CHAPTER 2.2.2, REFERENCES 52

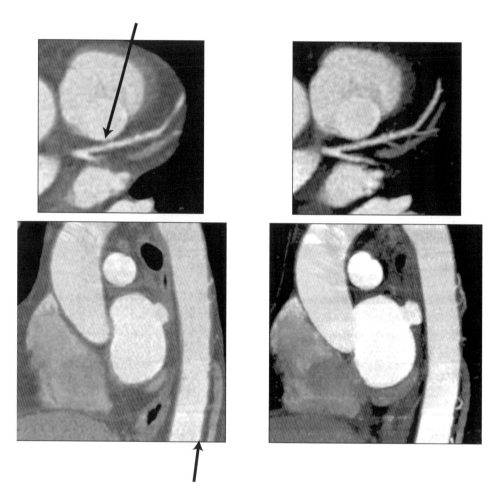

Figure 24 Multiplanar reconstruction (MPR) and maximum intensity projection (MIP)

Format: MPR, MIP (64-slice)

2-D images can be reconstructed in different formats at an arbitrary slice thickness. The simplest reconstruction method for visualization is the multiplanar reconstruction (MPR) (left panels). An MPR is a 2-D image displaying all pixels in a chosen plane. The original CT values are preserved. Therefore, in a contrast-enhanced image, for example of a coronary vessel, both the high-intensity signal of the contrast-filled lumen and the low-intensity signal of the vessel wall are represented. Another common reconstruction technique is the maximum intensity projection (MIP) (right panels). In contrast to the MPR, the MIP is a 2-D image displaying only the maximum intensity pixels. Therefore, in a contrast-enhanced MIP image of, for example, the coronary vessel, visualization of the lumen is optimized, but the wall structures are less well seen. Because of its similarity to conventional angiographic images, it is often used for CT angiography. However, only part of the original CT data are preserved, and findings should be confirmed on MPR images.

This figure shows images of a coronary artery and aorta in MPR and MIP modes. The normal vessel wall (arrows) is seen in the MPR images as a narrow rim surrounding the lumen.

CHAPTER 2.2.2, REFERENCES 52

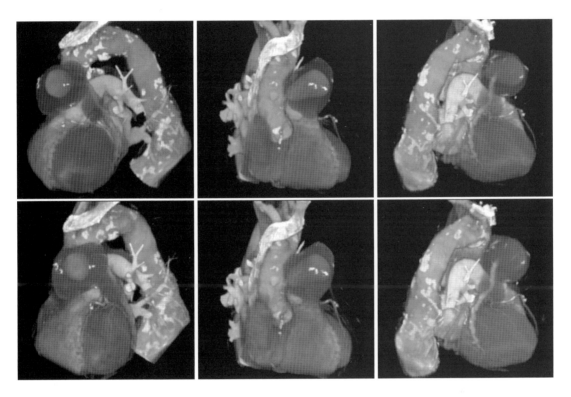

Figure 25   Volume-rendered image (VRI)

Format: VRI

Volume-rendered (VR) reconstruction employs advanced 3-D image processing algorithms with semitransparent visualization of superficial and deep contours. Each voxel is assigned a value for opacity according to its Hounsfield number, such that lower-intensity tissues are more transparent whereas higher-intensity tissues are more opaque. Therefore, the more opaque tissue is visible through translucent tissue, creating depth perception. VR images allow demonstration of complex anatomy and appreciation of the spatial relationship between visualized structures. Levels of opacity can be varied to alter the display of data as needed. In addition, the VR data can be viewed at arbitrary angles, including the standard views of conventional coronary angiography.

In this image several volume-rendered multidetector MDCT images of a coronary aneurysm at the origin of an aorto-coronary bypass graft to the left circumflex coronary artery are shown (Movie 29).

CHAPTER 2.2.3, REFERENCES 52, 53

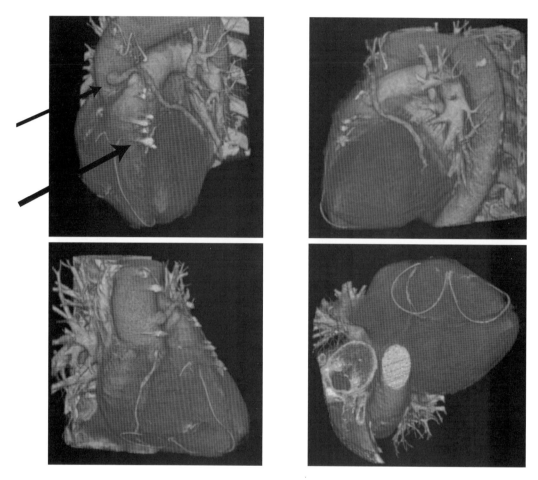

Figure 26 Color-coded VRI (see also color section on p. 5)

Format: VRI

VR images allow demonstration of complex anatomy and appreciation of the spatial relationship between visualized structures. Color-coding can also be used further to enhance the 3-D appearance.

In this image a color VR image of an aorto-coronary bypass graft to the left circumflex coronary artery (LCX) is shown (thin arrow). Also shown is blooming artifact related to surgical clips along a coronary bypass graft (left internal mammary artery (LIMA graft)) to the LAD (thick arrow). The high-intensity signal originating from metallic material leads to a characteristic artifact, which often precludes assessment of adjacent structures (e.g. coronary artery). Characteristically, the artifact is larger than the structure ('blooming'), because even a small area of high intensity increases the Hounsfield unit of the overall voxel, represented on the CT image.

CHAPTER 2.2.3, REFERENCES 52, 53

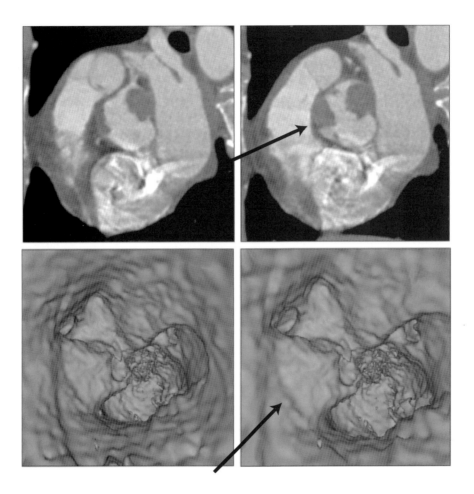

Figure 27   Perspective volume rendering (see also color section on p. 6)

Format: VRI, MPR

Perspective volume rendering (pVR) provides a virtual endoscopic view of the surface of anatomic structures that is sufficiently contrasted from surrounding tissue. This technique is used to visualize cavities or tubular structures accessible to endoscopes (e.g. the colon or the bronchial tree). Although the clinical value is unclear, it can also be applied to chambers of the heart or vascular structures, which can be viewed from within by rendering blood transparent. Tubular structures such as the coronary arteries can be viewed with motion along a path simulating flight through the vessel.

In this figure pVR images (lower panel) of thickened aortic valve leaflets (arrows) are shown in comparison with MPR images (upper panel).

CHAPTER 2.2.3, REFERENCES 52–55

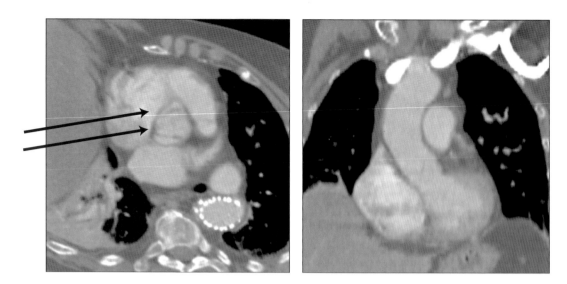

Figure 28 Motion artifact at aortic root

Format: MPR

Because of the rapid motion of the heart and the relatively long acquisition window, blurring of the image occurs, in particular if the acquisition window is not synchronized to the cardiac cycle. An important example is motion artifact at the root of the aorta in non-gated studies.

In this figure of a non-gated CT scan, image artifact at the aortic root is seen (arrows), which could be mistaken for a dissection flap. However, symmetry with linear structure on both sides of the aortic root is more typical for motion artifact.

CHAPTER 2.2.5.1, REFERENCE 58

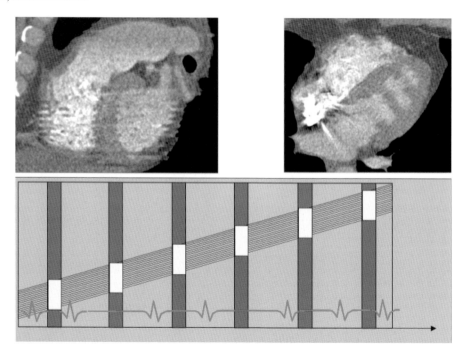

Figure 29 Arrhythmia artifact (1) (see also color section on p. 6)

Format: MPR, illustration

A typical artifact can be seen in patients with arrhythmia, and in particular atrial fibrillation. As shown in this figure, typical band-like shifts of the image data set are seen in image reconstructions. Each band represents the data obtained during one tube rotation and one heartbeat. Because data acquisition is performed at slightly different phases in subsequent cardiac cycles, the image stacks do not fit in the reconstruction.

CHAPTER 2.2.5.2, REFERENCES 58

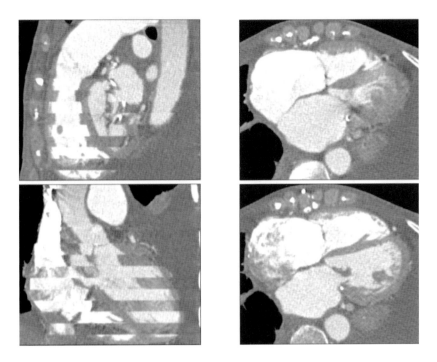

Figure 30   Arryhthmia artifact (2)

Format: MPR

Another example of the artifact caused by arrhythmia is shown in this figure. The typical band-like shifts of the image data set are more pronounced and thicker in these images from a 16-detector scanner.

CHAPTER 2.2.5.2, REFERENCES 58

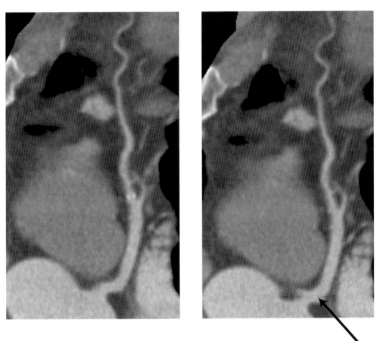

Figure 31   Arrhythmia artifact: extrasystole (1)

Format: MPR

A more subtle arrhythmia artifact occurs with individual extra beats. The images in this figure show misregistration in the proximal left main coronary artery (arrow). Modern CT systems allow editing of information from individual beats.

CHAPTER 2.2.5.2, REFERENCES 58

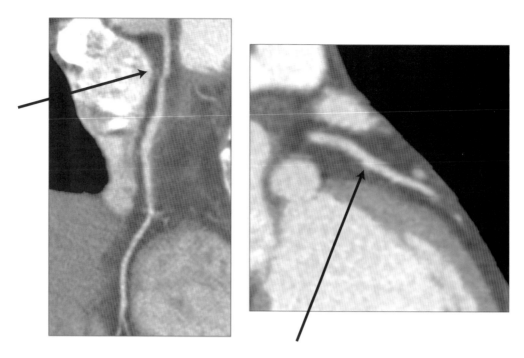

Figure 32   Arrhythmia artifact: extrasystole (2)

Format: MPR

Another example of this artifact in the proximal LAD is shown in this figure (arrows).

CHAPTER 2.2.5.2, REFERENCES 58

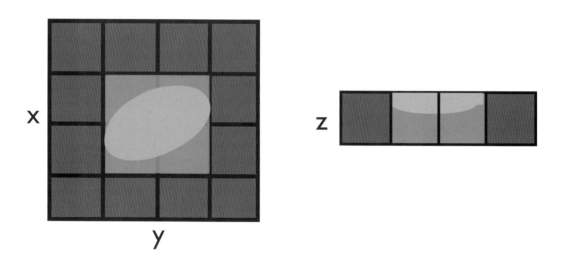

Figure 33   Partial volume averaging: blooming artifact (see also color section on p. 7)

Format: illustration

This figure illustrates partial volume averaging. It is not possible to resolve an object smaller than the voxel size. Although the oval object in this figure is smaller than the voxel size, the object is displayed with a size equal to the entire voxel volume (indicated by shaded volume). Therefore the object size is overestimated. This is called partial volume averaging or 'blooming' artifact.

CHAPTER 2.2.5.3, REFERENCES 58, 60

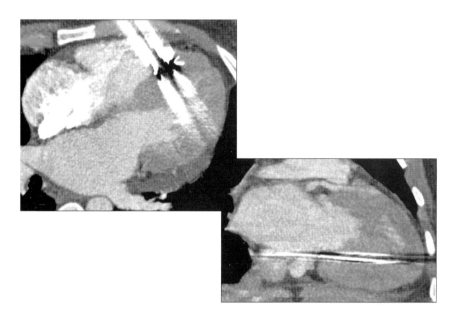

Figure 34   Streak artifact: metallic implants

Format: MPR

Larger areas of high-density material, in particular metallic foreign bodies, can severely reduce X-ray transmission. In the extreme, the detector may not record any signal transmission, causing the reconstruction algorithm to fail and produce streaks in the image originating from the source object. This has implications for cardiovascular imaging, as metal implants are common. Examples are pacer/implantable cardioverter defibrillator (ICD) wires, endovascular stents and surgical material.

The metal lead of pacer/ICD wires causes a strong artifact, which often precludes precise assessment of position, as shown in this image.

CHAPTER 2.2.5.4, REFERENCES 58, 60

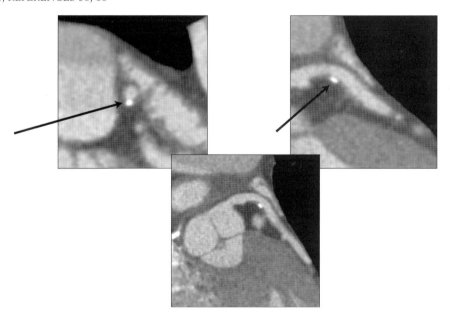

Figure 35   Blooming artifact: calcium

Format: MPR (64-slice)

This figure shows longitudinal and cross-sectional images of an LAD coronary artery obtained with a 64-slice system. The blooming artifact (arrows) of the calcified plaque in the mid-LAD segment is decreased in comparison with older CT systems. This appears to allow better differentiation between lumen and plaque.

CHAPTER 2.2.5.3, REFERENCES 58–60

3

The normal heart

Because of the oblique position of the cardiovascular structures in the chest (Figure 36), cardiovascular imaging relies on defined image planes oblique to the body axes. In contrast to axial images, imaging in planes along the organ axes avoids foreshortening (Figures 18 and 19). The following paragraph and the accompanying images introduce the most common standard oblique planes used to visualize cardiac structures. The left and right ventricles are typically visualized in oblique two-chamber, three-chamber, four-chamber and short-axis views (Figure 37) (Movies 6–9). The two-chamber view is comparable to the right anterior oblique (RAO) ventriculogram performed during angiography (Figure 38) (Movie 6). In contrast to angiography, CT and MRI visualize both the contrast-filled ventricular cavity and the myocardial wall. The three-chamber view includes the left atrium, left ventricle and aortic root, and is the basis to obtain additional images of the ascending aorta, demonstrating the anatomy of the aortic valve and aortic root (Figure 39). Beyond the aortic valve level, there is mild physiologic bulging in the area of the sinuses of Valsalva. The sinuses correspond to the three aortic valve cusps, including the non-coronary cusp (the cusp originating between left and right atria), and the right and left coronary cusps with the origin of the corresponding coronary arteries (Figure 40). The segment between the sinuses of Valsalva and the ascending aorta is called the sinotubular junction and typically causes a mild waist.

The standard display of coronary anatomy with conventional angiography includes views described by the position of the X-ray tube in relation to the patient. Standard views are, for example, right anterior oblique (RAO 30°), left anterior oblique (LAO 60°), etc. Volume-rendered images allow visualization of the course of the coronary arteries in relation to underlying cardiac chambers corresponding to the angiographic planes (Figures 41–44). However, the complex anatomy of coronary arteries is best assessed in multiple MPR and MIP images[50]. (see Chapter 4.1.2) (Figure 45) (Movie 10).

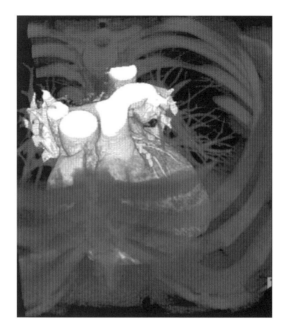

Figure 36 Heart in chest

Format: VRI

Because of the oblique position of the cardiovascular structures in the chest, cardiovascular imaging relies on defined image planes oblique to the body axes. In contrast to axial images, imaging in planes along the organ axes avoids foreshortening. This figure shows a volume-rendered image of the heart in the chest, demonstrating the oblique position, oblique to the axial scan orientation.

CHAPTER 3, REFERENCES 61–63

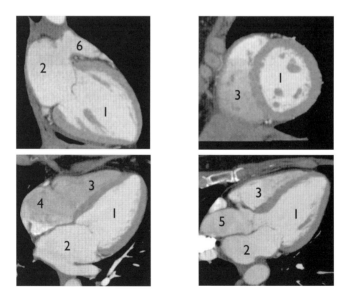

Figure 37 Standard views of cardiac chambers

Format: MPR

The left and right ventricles are typically visualized in oblique two-chamber, three-chamber, four-chamber and short-axis views.

Two-chamber (left upper panel), three-chamber (right lower panel), four-chamber (left lower panel) and short-axis (right upper panel) views of the ventricles are shown: 1, left ventricle; 2, left atrium; 3, right ventricle; 4, right atrium; 5, aortic root; 6, left atrial appendage.

CHAPTER 3, REFERENCES 61–63

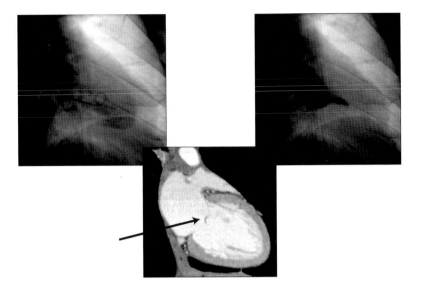

Figure 38 Two-chamber view in comparison with left ventriculogram

Format: MPR, angiography

The two-chamber view is comparable to the left ventriculogram in the right anterior oblique (RAO) projection, performed during angiography. In this figure a CT two-chamber view of the left ventricle (lower panel) is shown in comparison with the diastolic (left upper) and systolic (right upper) images from angiographic ventriculography. In contrast to angiography, which shows the contrast-filled ventricle, CT visualizes both the contrast-filled ventricular cavity and the myocardial wall. The CT images also visualize the mitral valve leaflets (arrow).

CHAPTER 3, REFERENCES 61–63

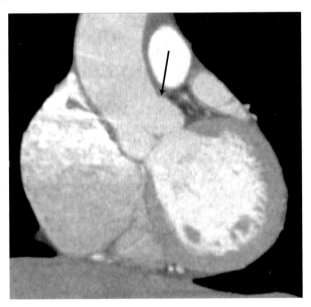

Figure 39 Aortic root

Format: MPR

This figure shows a normal aortic root and aortic valve. Beyond the valve level, there is mild physiologic bulging in the area of the sinuses of Valsalva. The sinuses correspond to the three aortic valve cusps, including the non-coronary cusp (the cusp originating in the area between left and right atria) and the right and left coronary cusps with the origin of the corresponding coronary arteries. The segment between the sinuses of Valsalva and the ascending aorta is called the sinotubular junction and typically causes a mild waist (arrow).

CHAPTER 3, REFERENCES 61–63

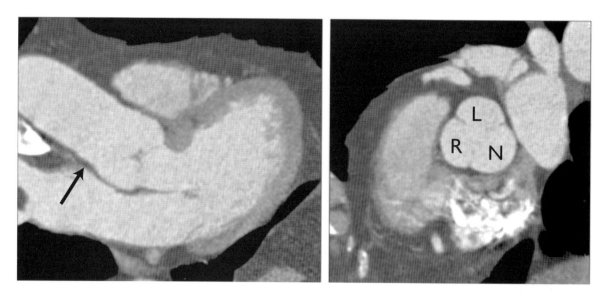

Figure 40   Normal tricuspid aortic valve

Format: MPR

This figure shows images of a tricuspid aortic valve. The short axis through the valve level (right panel) shows the three sinuses of Valsalva (N, non-coronary sinus, between left and right atria; L, left and R, right coronary sinus). There is mild prominence of the aortic root with mild effacement of the sinotubular junction (arrow).

CHAPTER 3, REFERENCES 61–63

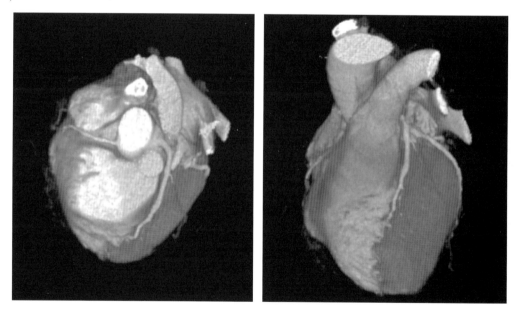

Figure 41   Left anterior oblique (LAO) view of coronary arteries

Format: VRI

The standard display of coronary anatomy with conventional angiography includes views described by the position of the X-ray tube in relation to the patient. Standard views are, for example, right anterior oblique (RAO 30°), left anterior oblique (LAO 60°), etc. Volume-rendered images allow the course of the coronary arteries to be shown in relation to underlying cardiac chambers corresponding to the angiographic planes. However, the complex anatomy of coronary arteries is best assessed in multiple MPR and MIP (see Chapter 4.1.2)

A VRI image of the heart with the left coronary arteries corresponding to LAO 60° views is shown (right panel). These VRI images provide an overall impression of coronary anatomy. However, findings on such images are typically confirmed on axial and oblique MPR and MIP images (see Chapter 4.1.2)

CHAPTER 3, REFERENCES 50, 61–63

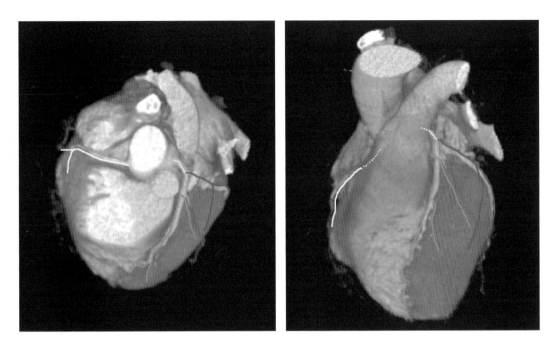

Figure 42 LAO view of coronary arteries (see also color section on p. 7)

Format: illustrated VRI

The same image as Figure 41 is shown with illustration of the course of the three coronary arteries. The left main coronary artery (LM) is shown in green, the left anterior descending coronary artery (LAD) in red, the left circumflex coronary artery (LCX) in green and the right coronary artery (RCA) in yellow.

CHAPTER 3, REFERENCES 50, 61–63

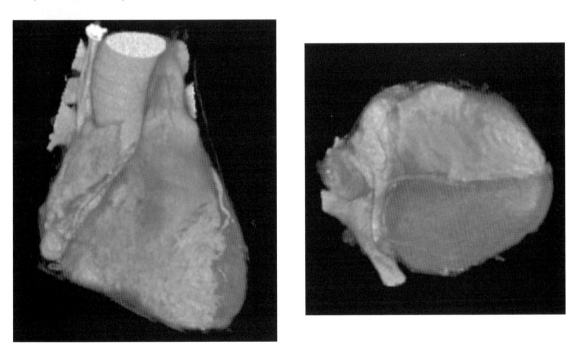

Figure 43 Right anterior oblique (RAO) views of coronary arteries

Format: VRI

A VRI image of the heart with the right coronary arteries corresponding to RAO 30° view (left panel) and from the inferior aspect of the heart (right panel) is shown.

CHAPTER 3, REFERENCES 50, 61–63

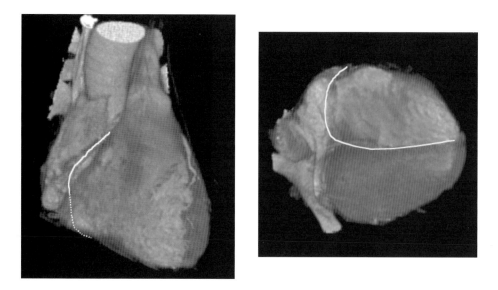

Figure 44   RAO view of coronary arteries (see also color section on p. 8)

Format: illustrated VRI

The same image as Figure 43 is shown with illustration of the course of the RCA.

CHAPTER 3, REFERENCES 50, 61–63

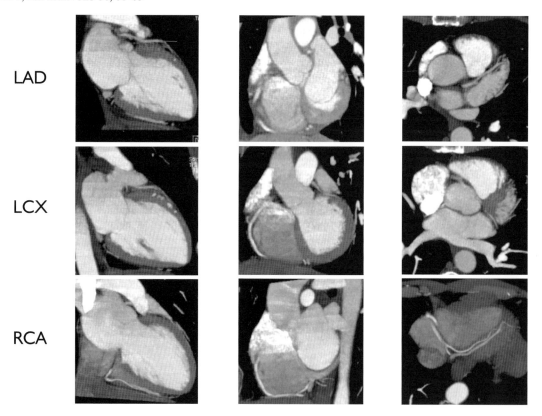

LAD

LCX

RCA

Figure 45   Coronary visualization with CT

Format: MPR

Volume-rendered images allow the course of the coronary arteries to be shown in relation to underlying cardiac chambers corresponding to the angiographic planes. However, the complex anatomy of coronary arteries is best assessed in multiple MPR and MIP (see Chapter 4.1.2)

In this figure, different segments of the three coronary arteries are shown.

CHAPTER 3, REFERENCES 50, 61–63

4

Clinical cardiovascular applications

Imaging is an essential part of the diagnostic work-up of patients with cardiovascular diseases. In clinical cardiology, a presumptive diagnosis is typically formed based on the physical examination and history, and the most appropriate imaging modality is then chosen to confirm or refute this diagnosis. Systematic textbooks of cardiovascular medicine[61,62] provide this clinical perspective for the interested reader.

The clinical chapters and the accompanying images in the atlas describe the expanding experience with MDCT for common and more unusual clinical cardiovascular indications. However, the chapters of the manual are not intended to provide a comprehensive description of imaging of cardiovascular disease.

4.1 ACQUIRED CARDIOVASCULAR DISEASES

4.1.1 Cardiac chambers and myocardium

Contrast-enhanced CT provides detailed anatomic information about the cardiac chambers and the myocardium. The high spatial resolution and the ability to reconstruct along oblique axes allow assessment of global and focal myocardial pathology. CT can therefore provide useful information in patients with non-ischemic and ischemic cardiomyopathies. However, in the assessment of these conditions, functional assessment of ventricular function and integrity of the valvular structures is essential. This functional assessment is a strength of echocardiography[63] and MRI[64], which therefore are typically the initial diagnostic tests performed in the

work-up of these patients. CT is performed if morphologic findings are in question. More recently, limited functional assessment has become possible with CT by combining multiple image reconstructions from different phases of the cardiac cycle into a cine-loop (Movies 1, 2, and 5). The clinical role of assessing function with CT is currently being evaluated. In the assessment of left ventricular (LV) measurements with MDCT, previous studies show a good correlation of the left ventricular ejection fraction (LVEF) values with cine-MRI, but significant underestimation of LV volumes with MDCT[57] (Figure 46).

The following paragraphs describe typical CT findings in patients with myocardial disease.

4.1.1.1 Non-ischemic cardiomyopathies

Dilated cardiomyopathy (DCM) The typical findings in patients with dilated cardiomyopathy are ventricular dilatation with relative thinning of the myocardium[65,66] (Figure 47). These findings can involve the left and right ventricles and are associated with ventricular dysfunction of various degrees.

In contrast to patients with ischemic cardiomyopathy, the coronary arteries are typically normal or only mildly diseased. Therefore, in the initial clinical assessment of these patients, who present with non-specific symptoms of heart failure, an assessment of coronary anatomy is typically performed with conventional angiography. The role of non-invasive angiography with MDCT is currently being evaluated.

Hypertrophic cardiomyopathy (HCM) and hypertrophic obstructive cardiomyopathy (HOCM) This group of cardiomyopathies is characterized by primary myocardial hypertrophy. Different entities have characteristic distributions of the hypertrophic myocardium. Apical HCM (Yamaguchi) is characterized by concentric left ventricular thickening in the distal and apical left ventricular segments (Figures 48–50). The classic morphologic finding in patients with hypertrophic obstructive cardiomyopathy (HOCM) is asymmetric septal hypertrophy[65,67] (Figure 51). However, functional evidence of outflow tract obstruction (typically assessed with echocardiography) is necessary for the diagnosis. Non-obstructive hypertrophic cardiomyopathy is differentiated by the absence of outflow tract obstruction (Figure 52).

Restrictive cardiomyopathy (RCM) Restrictive cardiomyopathies are a group of disease conditions characterized by increased ventricular stiffness. A diagnostic hallmark is diastolic dysfunction, which is best assessed with echocardiography[63,65,68]. Ventricular stiffness can be secondary to myocardial infiltration (e.g. cardiac amyloidosis), where advanced disease stages potentially show myocardial prominence and can involve both the left and right ventricular wall (Figure 53). Alternatively, restriction can be caused by endocardial fibrosis (e.g. Loeffler's endocarditis) (Figure 54) (Movies 11 and 12).

Arrhythmogenic right ventricular dysplasia (ARVD) Arrhythmogenic right ventricular dysplasia describes a clinical syndrome of life-threatening ventricular tachycardia, originating from foci of a remodeled right ventricular wall. Major and minor diagnostic criteria have been described[69,70]. Major imaging criteria are global right ventricular dysfunction, global right ventricular cavity dilatation, and focal right ventricular wall aneurysm formation (Figure 55). Minor imaging criteria are focal wall thinning with fibrous or fatty replacement of myocardium involving the right ventricular and sometimes the left ventricular myocardium[71–73] (Figures 55–58).

The major, functional criteria are best assessed with MRI. However, because of better spatial resolution, MDCT offers advantages in characterizing myocardial wall abnormalities, including thinning, focal aneurysm formation, and fatty or fibrous replacement (Figures 55–58). Recent advances in the dynamic reconstruction of spiral data allow visualization of right ventricular wall motion. However, experience is still limited.

4.1.1.2 Non-ischemic atrial and ventricular aneurysms and diverticula

Left ventricular diverticula are small, congenital outpouchings of the left ventricular cavity with maintained wall structure (Figures 59 and 60). Diverticula can be differentiated from focal aneurysms by the maintained contractility on functional studies (Movies 13 and 14).

Aneurysmal bulging of the intra-atrial septum and fibrous part of the intraventricular septum can be visualized with CT (Figures 61 and 62). However, further assessment of shunt flow requires examination with echocardiography and MRI.

4.1.1.3 Ischemic cardiomyopathy

Acute coronary syndromes The clinical approach to patients presenting with high likelihood of an acute coronary syndrome is based on the emergent, early assessment of coronary anatomy in order to decide about revascularization[74]. Because of its reliable definition of highly stenotic lesions and the opportunity for immediate therapeutic intervention, conventional angiography remains the test of choice in the acute setting[74].

Animal models and occasional clinical observations describe areas of decreased contrast enhancement in hypoperfused myocardial segments[75–78]. However, it is currently not completely understood if these findings differentiate between acute or chronic changes (Figures 63 and 64), and comparison with delayed contrast-enhancement MRI[79] has not been performed.

CT has an established role in the evaluation of subacute complications of acute myocardial infarction, including free wall rupture and pseudoaneurysm formation[80,81] (Figure 65) (Movies 15–17).

Chronic ischemic cardiomyopathy Areas of remote left ventricular myocardial infarction typically demonstrate ventricular wall thinning with fibrous or calcified replacement of myocardium, and aneurysm formation with or without cavitary thrombus (Figures 66–72) (Movies 18 and 19). Focal aneurysms can be differentiated from diverticula by the lack of contraction on functional studies (see Chapter 4.1.1.2).

4.1.1.4 Atrial and ventricular thrombus formation

Atrial and ventricular thrombus formation is associated with various underlying pathologies. Left atrial appendage (LAA) clot is common and frequently associated with atrial fibrillation. It appears as a filling defect in the appendage (Figures 73 and 74). However, slow flow in the left atrial appendage as described by transesophageal echocardiography[82,83] may appear as an LAA filling defect on CT. LAA filling may also depend on contrast timing. Right atrial thrombus is less common, and underlying abnormalities of coagulation are often suspected (Figure 75).

Left ventricular thrombus is often associated with post-infarct aneurysms (Figure 70). Occasional left ventricular clot without underlying dysfunction is found (Figure 76).

Unusual findings are atrial or ventricular wall hematoma after open-heart surgery (Figures 77 and 78).

4.1.1.5 Other findings of the ventricles

Left ventricular non-compaction describes an incidental finding of prominent left ventricular trabeculation, related to embryonic wall development[84,85] (Figures 79–81) (Movies 20–22).

Lipomatous hypertrophy describes prominent fatty infiltration of the intra-atrial septum[86,87] (Figure 82).

An unusual finding is myocardial scar secondary to myocarditis (Figure 83). In contrast to scar related to coronary artery disease (CAD), the distribution of the scar tissue does not follow vascular territories and is often more focal[88]. Similarly, focal scar formation not following vascular distribution is seen in cardiac sarcoidosis (Figure 84).

A postoperative pseudoaneurysm of the left ventricle originating at the mitral annulus in a patient with remote mitral valve surgery is shown in Figure 85.

An anecdotal finding is illustrated in Figure 86, showing a fragment of an injection needle trapped in the apex of the right ventricle.

4.1.2 Atherosclerotic coronary artery disease

Modern CT imaging provides a comprehensive assessment of coronary anatomy[27,89–92] (Figures 87–89). Non-contrast-enhanced scans (CT calcium scoring) allow an assessment of calcified plaque burden. Indications for contrast-enhanced protocols (CT angiography, CTA) are the evaluation of arterial stenosis, bypass grafts and stents. CTA is also applied to the assessment of non-atherosclerotic CAD, such as coronary anomalies, coronary muscle bridge and coronary aneurysm. In addition, novel applications include the evaluation of subclinical atherosclerosis.

Emphasizing the ability of CT for a comprehensive assessment of different stages of CAD, the following sections describe early atherosclerotic changes and more advanced stenotic stages.

4.1.2.1 Non-stenotic, subclinical CAD

Atherosclerotic plaque accumulation in the vessel wall begins long before the development of angiographic stenosis[93–95]. In fact, it is now well known that most acute coronary events are initiated by rupture or erosion of mildly stenotic but vulnerable (high-risk) lesions[96,97]. Modern atherosclerosis imaging is therefore evaluating overall plaque burden and plaque characteristics as predictors of future cardiovascular risk. Non-enhanced CT imaging (CT calcium scoring) allows the assessment of calcified plaque, whereas contrast-enhanced CTA allows differentiation of calcified and non-calcified plaque.

Calcium scoring The identification of coronary arterial calcification is a reliable sign of chronic atherosclerotic changes. Advanced stenotic lesions causing chronic, stable angina pectoris often demonstrate dense calcifications. In contrast, high-risk culprit lesions causing acute coronary events are frequently non-calcified or show microcalcification on histology[98,99]. CT examinations performed without contrast administration are very sensitive in detecting and quantifying coronary arterial calcification[100,101] (Figures 90 and 91). The prevalence of coronary calcification is higher in men, and increases with age[102,103]. Total calcium load in the coronary tree can be quantified using one of several calcium scoring algorithms, including the traditional Agaston score[100], volume scoring[104] and mass scoring[105]. The initial experience with calcium scoring was gained with EBCT. MDCT has recently emerged as an alternative method for calcium detection and quantification[106–108]. Standardized scan and scoring protocols are currently being developed for MDCT calcium scoring using cross-technology calibration methods. Reproducibility in the detection and quantification of coronary artery calcium is critical to the establishment of MDCT as a valid method for calcium scoring[109–113]. Recently, the quantification of calcium from contrast-enhanced MDCT images has been proposed, using a threshold equal to 350 Hounsfield units (HU)[114].

Coronary calcium scores have been shown to correlate with the total atherosclerotic plaque burden (calcified and non-calcified plaque)[115,116], and the predictive value of the overall EBCT calcium score for future coronary events has been shown[117,118]. Dynamic changes in the calcium volume score during pharmacological therapy have been examined in serial CT studies[119,120]. Despite limited prospective data about the incremental value of calcium scores over 'traditional' multivariate risk-assessment models, the 2000 American Heart Association/American College of Cardiology (AHA/ACC) consensus statements concluded that calcium screening may be justified in selected patient groups with intermediate risk[121]. This hypothesis has been supported by data from recently published studies[122,123].

Contrast-enhanced CTA for plaque imaging Coronary calcium scores identify calcified plaque but significantly underestimate total atherosclerotic plaque burden (calcified and non-calcified plaque)[114,115]. Despite the predictive value of the overall EBCT calcium score for future coronary events the site of calcification does not localize the future event, because acute events may originate from non-calcified plaque (Figures 92 and 93).

Contrast-enhanced CT scans allow differentiation of lumen and vessel wall, and subsequently the identification of both calcified and non-calcified plaque[124–128]. Similar to the experience with intra-vascular ultrasound (IVUS)[129–133], emerging studies demonstrate the frequent presence of plaque burden in segments without luminal stenosis (Figures 94 to 99). These studies also demonstrate the association of plaque accumulation with outward expansion of the vessel wall (expansive remodeling), maintaining luminal dimension[127,134] (Figures 96 and 97). In recent studies, non-calcified plaque has been further characterized on the basis of mean Hounsfield number and compared with plaque characteristics by IVUS[124,126,135,136]. Typical results describe a density of < 50 HU for soft plaques, 50–120 HU for intermediate plaques and > 120 HU for calcified lesions with. Semi-automated software systems for plaque analysis are currently being evaluated. The rationale of these studies is that the identification of 'vulnerable' atherosclerotic lesions and the overall plaque burden could provide better markers of coronary risk than measures of luminal stenosis[137–141].

4.1.2.2 Stenotic, clinical CAD

Coronary CT angiography (CTA) Challenges for coronary CT angiography (CTA) are the small size of coronary arteries, the tortuous course and the fast motion during the cardiac cycle[142–149]. Large coronary segments with minimal motion, e.g. the left main coronary artery (LM) and proximal portions of the left anterior descending artery (LAD), are more reliably visualized than segments with more pronounced motion, including parts of the right coronary artery (RCA) and circumflex coronary artery (LCX), and smaller segments. Coronary arterial motion varies during the cardiac cycle, and individual arteries reach peak velocity at different times during the cycle[150]. Therefore, to assess optimally all coronary arteries in one patient, image reconstruction is often performed at several phases in the cardiac cycle[30,31] (Figure 10). The best image quality with 500-ms rotation scanners is usually achieved at 50–70% of the RR interval for the LAD, 50–60% for the LCX and 40–50% for the RCA. However, owing to considerable interpatient variation, evaluation at various phases in the cardiac cycle is recommended for optimization of reconstruction on a patient-by-patient basis.

Another important limitation of CTA is related to coronary arterial calcification. The 'blooming' (or 'volume average') effect of coronary calcification can result in potential false-positive detection or overestimation of luminal stenosis, and can cause difficulties in assessing adjacent non-calcified plaque structures[147] (Figures 98–100). Advances in scanner technology are expected to reduce this artifact (Figures 8 and 35). Consistent with these limitations, CT angiography has been shown to have a high negative predictive value in the exclusion of severe stenosis but a lower positive predictive value for the detection of severe luminal stenosis, in comparison with X-ray angiography[147,148,151]. Sensitivities ranging from 75 to 85% and specificities from 76 to 99% were reported for the assessment of coronary stenoses > 50%. Recent studies using 16-slice systems report improved visualization with a lower percentage of poorly assessable segments and higher sensitivity and specificity[152,153] (Figures 98–110). The potential value of CT in assessing perfusion defects associated with severe luminal stenosis is discussed in Chapter 4.1.1.3 (Figures 63 and 64).

Because of the high negative predictive value, CTA may be suitable for clinical situations in which exclusion of significant proximal disease is required.

This could include preoperative coronary evaluation before non-cardiac surgery.

CT may also provide complementary information for subgroups of significant lesions, including pre-interventional assessment of lesion calcification and assessment of unclear left main coronary artery lesions (Figures 111–119) (Movies 23 and 24).

Non-stenotic forms of atherosclerotic disease, including diffuse coronary ectasia and aneurysms, can be evaluated with MDCT[154] (Figures 120–126). Non-atherosclerotic aneurysms must be differentiated (Figure 127) (Movie 25). Coronary anomalies are described in Chapter 4.2.2.

CTA has documented value for surveillance after coronary revascularization. Graft patency can be assessed in surgical bypass grafts. Because of their relatively large size compared to internal mammary grafts, venous aorto-coronary grafts can also be evaluated for the presence and severity of stenosis[155–159] (Figures 128–141) (Movies 26–30). When assessing bypass grafts, artifact from metallic surgical clips often obscures the adjacent portion of a coronary graft, a common situation for internal mammary grafts (Figure 26). Because of their large size, stents in bypass grafts can be assessed (Figures 132 and 133). Unusual findings, including graft aneurysms, can be described (Figures 134–139) (Movie 29). An important application is the assessment of graft position before repeat bypass surgery, to avoid injury during surgery[160] (Figures 140 and 141) (Movie 30).

The high-density metallic mesh of coronary stents precludes confident detection and grading of in-stent restenosis with CT. However, differentiation between stent patency and occlusion and evaluation of stenosis at the leading or trailing ends of a stent are often possible[161–163] (Figures 142–145). When inferring stent patency from the presence of luminal enhancement distal to the stent, it is important to note that retrograde filling from collaterals cannot be differentiated by CT. Improved stent visualization is expected with higher in-plane spatial resolution of recently introduced CT scanners.

4.1.3 Coronary veins and coronary sinus

Because of the peripheral intravenous rather than selective arterial contrast injection, the coronary sinus and coronary veins are typically slightly contrast enhanced on CT images[164,165]. Segments of the coronary veins are parallel to the course of the coronary arteries and can therefore be mistaken for coronary arteries. If the venous structures are the primary focus of the examination, slightly different contrast timing or multiphasic imaging is often performed (Figure 146). An emerging clinical question is assessment of the coronary sinus anatomy for placement of biventricular pacer leads (Figure 147). Unusual coronary sinus findings include coronary sinus/left atrial fistula (Figure 148).

4.1.4 Pericardial disease

Normal pericardial anatomy is characterized by layers of fat on the epicardial and pericardial surfaces of the heart which provide natural contrast, permitting reliable identification of pericardium on non-contrast-enhanced CT scans[166–168]. CT scans after contrast administration are preferred because additional information, including evidence of inflammation with pericardial enhancement, can be obtained. The normal pericardium, which has a thickness of 1–2 mm, can be delineated over the left and right ventricles (Figures 149 and 150) (Movie 31). Congenital or postsurgical absence of the pericardium (Figures 151–157), pericardial thickening (Figures 158 and 159) and pericardial calcification (Figures 159–164) can be reliably identified. The detection of increased pericardial thickness, especially with pericardial calcium, in combination with conical/tubular deformation of the ventricles, provides evidence of pericardial constriction (Figure 165). However, these findings do not prove the presence of constrictive physiology, which is best assessed with echocardiography or MRI (Figure 166). The recent introduction of 4-D CT software allows functional assessment, but experience is limited (Movie 32). As described above, pericardial enhancement after contrast injection is consistent with pericarditis (Figures 167–169).

CT allows reliable identification of pericardial effusion adjacent to the left and right ventricles and quantification of the amount and characteristics of pericardial fluid (Figures 170 and 171). Findings consistent with tamponade are right ventricular collapse or indirect signs including enlargement of the hepatic veins (Figure 172). However, a functional assessment of tamponade physiology is the strength of echocardiography and MRI.

Pericardial cysts (Figures 173 and 174) and primary or metastatic pericardial tumors (Chapter 4.1.5) can be defined in relation to adjacent structures.

4.1.5 Cardiac masses

Cardiac masses can be described with regard to size, density, contrast enhancement and spatial relationship to adjacent structures[169]. However, the morphology of tumors is highly variable, and qualitative assessment with CT is limited. Because of its superior tissue characterization, MRI often allows further qualitative classification and should be considered complementary[169,170]. A frequent clinical question is the differentiation between benign and malignant processes. Imaging can provide important clues, but the definitive diagnosis requires surgical sampling and pathology. The following examples of benign and malignant tumors demonstrate basic imaging criteria.

Common benign tumors are atrial myxomas. Myxomas often originate from the left atrium or mitral annulus with a stalk, and may demonstrate tumor calcification (Figures 175 and 176). 4-D imaging allows assessment of mobility (Figure 177) (Movies 1 and 2). However, definitive characterization is often not possible with CT imaging alone (Figures 178–180) (Movies 33 and 34). Follow-up imaging demonstrating stability of findings over time is confirmation of the likely benign nature of masses (Figure 181). Benign masses of the left ventricle have similar characteristics. Additional MRI imaging is often utilized for further characterization (Figures 182 and 183).

There is a wide variety of primary and secondary malignant cardiac tumors. Signs of malignancy which can be assessed with CT include infiltration of adjacent structures and the presence of tumor vessels. Examples are shown in the corresponding figures (Figures 184–193) (Movies 35–38).

4.1.6 Valvular heart disease

The assessment of valvular heart disease is a strength of magnetic resonance imaging, and in particular echocardiography. Imaging of valvular structures with CT is limited owing to the minimal thickness and significant motion during the cardiac cycle[65,171] (Figures 194–196). Advances in scanner technology are likely to improve assessment of valvular structures (Figure 7). Imaging of the aortic valve allows differentiation between normal tricuspid (Figure 40) and abnormal bicuspid (Figures 197–201) aortic valve anatomy. CT can precisely describe the extent and location of valvular calcification, for example in patients with aortic stenosis (Figure 202).

Similarly, thickening and calcification of the mitral valve leaflets, which is often associated with mitral stenosis, can be described (Figure 203). The typical systolic displacement of the mitral valve leaflets can be demonstrated in patients with mitral valve prolapse (Figure 204). In patients with Ebstein's anomaly the displacement of the tricuspid valve towards the right ventricle can be seen (Figure 205).

Thickening of the valve leaflets and tissue adjacent to the valves can be assessed (Figures 206–208). However, reliable assessment of vegetations remains a strength of echocardiography.

A strength of CT is the postoperative evaluation after valve replacement. Correct position of the prosthetic valve can be assessed (Figures 209–214), and complications including valve dehiscence identified (Figure 215).

4.1.7 Aortic disease

MDCT imaging of the aorta has become the diagnostic standard for a wide range of acute and chronic clinical indications, including aortic aneurysms, aortic dissections, intramural hematomas and endovascular stent imaging[172,173]. Contrast enhancement is crucial for most indications to differentiate the lumen and the vessel wall.

With four-slice scanners, spiral scans without ECG referencing were typically used to image the entire thoracic aorta. Additional ECG-gated acquisitions were performed to cover the ascending aorta in order reduce motion artifact of the aortic root and ascending aorta[174,175] (Figure 28). In contrast, the speed of modern multidetector scanners allows scanning of the entire thoracic and abdominal aorta in one breath-hold with standard retrospective ECG-gated spiral techniques.

In the assessment of aortic dissections, an important aspect is the involvement of the ascending aorta. Type-A dissections, which involve the ascending aorta, are typically operated immediately[176] (Figures 216 and 217). The identification of acute complications, in particular rupture and hemoperitoneum and hemopericardium, is crucial in the clinical assessment of these patients (Figures 218 and 219). Type-B dissections, which begin beyond the origin of the left subclavian artery, are often treated medically. However, complications including visceral branch vessel compression and rupture can require immediate treatment (Figures 220 and 221). The location of non-communicating intramural hematomas can be described in analogy to communicating dissections[177,178] (Figures 222–224). Because of the high spatial resolution of modern scanners, allowing detailed characterization of the vessel wall, CT imaging is the preferred modality for intramural hematomas (Figures 225 and 226). The clinical significance of large penetrating ulcerations is less well defined[179] (Figure 227). Leakage of an aneurysm can be seen in acute situations (Figure 228).

CT is routinely performed for the identification of thoracic and abdominal aortic aneurysms. Reconstruction of images perpendicular to the vessel axis for each segment of the aorta allows precise assessment and measurement of aneurysms of the sinuses of Valsalva (Figures 229 and 230) (Movies 39–41), ectasia of the aortic root and ascending aorta (Figures 231–234), atherosclerotic and post-traumatic aneurysms of the descending thoracic aorta (Figures 235–237) and aneurysms of the abdominal aorta. If an aortic dissection is super-imposed on an existing aneurysm, the dissection typically ends proximal to or at the level of the aneurysm. However, occasionally the dissection extends beyond the area of the aneurysm (Figure 238).

An important application of CT is perioperative imaging of the aorta in patients undergoing cardiac and aortic surgery. In patients undergoing open heart surgery, the local extent of calcified atherosclerotic plaque can determine the cannulation site during cardiopulmonary bypass. To assess the amount of calcification, a non-contrast-enhanced CT scan is performed (Figures 239 and 240). Contrast-enhanced scans can assess the amount of calcified and non-calcified atherosclerotic plaque, which is related to postoperative stroke incidence[180,181] (Figure 241). Similarly, preoperative CT can help in planning the surgical access site in patients with thoracoabdominal aneurysm (Figure 242).

Postoperative CT scans are useful in the assessment of surgical results (Figures 243–246) (Movies 42 and 43) and early and late complications. In the early postoperative phase, complications at the repair site or in the operative field, including mediastinal hematoma or infection (Figures 247 and 248), pericardial or pleural effusion and pneumo-thorax, can be identified. Late complications include prosthetic valve graft infections, postoperative

pseudoaneurysms and fistulas after surgery (Figures 249–258).

CT imaging of the aorta is an integral part of endovascular stent graft therapy of aortic aneurysms[182–185] (Figures 259 and 260). Three-dimensional reconstructions of diseased aortic segments are used for precise quantitative assessment of custom-made stent grafts[186].

Morphologic changes associated with aortitis in the context of connective-tissue diseases can be assessed with CT. Typical findings are wall thickening and extensive calcification in later stages (Figure 240). The potential role of positron emission tomography (PET)/CT scanners for the assessment of disease activity is currently being evaluated (Figure 261).

An incidental finding of an intra-aortic balloon pump in the aorta is shown in Figure 262. Aortic coarctation is described in the section below on congenital disease (Chapter 4.2.6).

4.1.8 Pulmonary circulation

4.1.8.1 Pulmonary artery

Contrast-enhanced CT has a high sensitivity and specificity for the diagnosis of proximal pulmonary embolus (main through-segmental arteries) in comparison to ventilation–perfusion (VQ) scans[187–191] (Figure 263). The advantages of CT are the speed and wide availability in many emergency departments. The CT scan allows direct visualization of the thrombus, and simultaneous assessment of the lung parenchyma and size of the cardiac chambers (e.g. right ventricular enlargement). An extension of the scan through the abdomen and pelvis has been performed to identify the source of the embolus[192]. CT does not provide an assessment of lung ventilation or perfusion (VQ scan) or right ventricular function (echocardiography, MRI)[193].

An unusual finding is a pseudoaneurysm of the pulmonary artery (Figure 264).

4.1.8.2 Pulmonary veins

Historically, pulmonary vein anatomy was mainly relevant in the assessment of abnormal venous return as part of congenital syndromes (see Chapter 4.2.7.2). However, more recently, percutaneous ablation procedures at the pulmonary vein ostia have become a standard treatment for chronic atrial fibrillation in specialized clinical centers. Imaging of the pulmonary veins is now commonly performed before the procedure for 3-D guidance[194,195] (Figure 265) and after the procedure for diagnosis and surveillance of pulmonary vein stenosis[196,197]. In addition, the left atrium and left atrial appendage can be assessed for thrombus (Figures 73, 74 and 266). Post-interventional complications include wall thickening and luminal stenosis (Figures 266–271). CT is sensitive in identifying and grading stenosis but limited in differentiating subtotal and total venous occlusion (Figures 270 and 271). An important advantage of CT is the ability to visualize inflammatory changes associated with the development of vein stenosis, including wall thickening at the vein ostia and mediastinal lymph node enlargement (Figures 268 and 269). If severe pulmonary vein stenosis requires angioplasty and stenting, stent position and patency can be assessed with CT (Figures 272 and 273).

4.1.9 Peripheral arterial disease

Because of the larger size, lack of motion and straight course of peripheral arteries, the identification and quantification of luminal stenosis can be performed with CT angiography[198,199]. MDCT protocols use a spiral examination mode with thin, overlapping images. It is important to time the rapid contrast bolus injection carefully for arterial enhancement[44]. CT angiography has developed into an alternative imaging modality in several vascular regions. In neuroradiology, modern systems allow simultaneous imaging of the carotid arteries, intracranial vessels, brain morphology and brain perfusion[200]. CT angiography is also increasingly used for the assessment of renal artery disease, carotid disease and atherosclerotic disease of the lower-extremity arteries, often as a 'roadmap' for subsequent angioplasty[201–204]. A disadvantage of CT in comparison with ultrasound and MRI is the associated radiation exposure and the lack of flow information.

4.2 ADULT CONGENITAL HEART DISEASE

MDCT is increasingly used in pediatric patients as a second-line imaging modality after echocardiography and MRI, if anatomic findings are unclear or confirmation is required. Because of the short acquisition time, CT can frequently be performed with mild sedation (Figures 274–278). However, because of the radiation exposure, a particularly

careful evaluation of the risk and benefits is necessary in children. The interested reader is referred to the specialized literature[205,206].

Consistent with the overall purpose of the book, this chapter describes mainly congenital abnormalities which are seen in adults[207]. The description follows the order of the previous sections.

4.2.1 Cardiac chambers and myocardium

Atrial septal defects (ASD) are common congenital heart defects. The different types of defect (ostium secundum defect, ostium primum defect, sinus venosus defect, coronary sinus defect and patent foramen ovale (PFO)) are related to the embryonal development of the intra-atrial septum. Unrepaired defects are occasionally identified in asymptomatic or symptomatic adults. Symptoms can include right heart failure or neurologic symptoms secondary to paradoxical embolization. Because the central intra-atrial septum is a very thin structure, anatomic assessment with imaging modalities is limited. Identification of these defects typically relies on the assessment of flow by echocardiography and MRI (Movies 44 and 45). Anatomic assessment with CT can define the relationship of the defect to other anatomic structures, such as the coronary sinus (Figure 279) or the sinus venosus (Figure 280). Surgical or percutaneous closure of ASD is considered, depending on the clinical situation and anatomic characteristics. CT is increasingly being used for pre- and post-interventional imaging in the setting of percutaneous closure (Figure 281) (Movie 46).

Ventricular septal defects (VSD) are common in childhood, but either close spontaneously or are closed surgically early on. They are therefore less commonly seen in adults. The different types of VSD (perimembraneous VSD, muscular or apical VSD, inlet of atrioventricular canal VSD, supracristal or subaortic VSD) are related to the embryonal development of the interventricular septum. CT can identify the defect and describe the relationship to surrounding structures (Figures 282–284). Echocardiography, MRI and cardiac catheterization with evaluation of oxygen saturation, flow and pressure measurements are important for functional assessment.

Right ventricular dysplasia (ARVD) (Chapter 4.1.1.1), LV non-compaction (Chapter 4.1.1.5) and hypertrophic obstructive cardiomyopathy (HOCM) (Chapter 4.1.1.1) are described elsewhere.

4.2.2 Coronary arteries

The assessment of coronary anomalies is a strength of MDCT, in particular because of the facility for 3-D reconstruction[208,209]. Image reconstruction allows definition of the origin of anomalous arteries (compare with Figure 40).

Variants without clinical significance are seen, for example left main origin of the non-coronary instead of the left coronary cusp (Figures 285–287). More significant is the origin of the right or left coronary system from the contralateral cusp or artery (Figures 288–297) (Movie 47). The course of the anomalous artery as it crosses the midline determines the clinical significance. In some cases, the anomalous artery has a course posterior to the aortic root, between the aortic root and the left atrium (Figure 290). More commonly, the artery can take a course anterior to the aortic root (Figure 291). A low course, crossing between the aortic root and pulmonary outflow, is described as intracristal (Figures 292,293). A high course, crossing between the aorta and pulmonary artery, has a higher risk, because of possible systolic compression between the two structures (Figure 294). The demonstration of an anomalous course between the aorta and the pulmonary artery may therefore define an indication for surgical correction. An advantage of CT is description of the relationship of the anomalous coronary artery to other cardiovascular structures. This becomes obvious in cases of coronary fistulas (Figures 298–303) (Movie 48) and in the evaluation of an intramyocardial course of a coronary muscle bridge (Figure 304).

4.2.3 Coronary veins and coronary sinus

Images of a patient with a coronary sinus aneurysm are shown in Figure 305[210].

4.2.4 Pericardial disease

Images of patients with absence of the pericardium are shown in Figures 151–157.

4.2.5 Valvular heart disease

Images of a patient with Ebstein's anomaly of the tricuspid valve are shown in Figure 205.

4.2.6 Aortic disease

CT can demonstrate the anatomy of unrepaired aortic coarctation[211] (Figures 306 and 307) and results after percutanous (Figures 308 amd 309) and surgical (Figures 310 and 311) repair. The known association with bicuspid aortic valve should be considered (Figures 306 and 309). Images of a patient with evidence of surgical repair after an interrupted aortic arch are shown in Figure 312.

Marfan's syndrome (Figures 233 and 234) is a multisystem connective-tissue disorder associated with a mutation in the fibrillin (*FBN*1) gene. There is an association with aortic root dilatation and subsequent regurgitation, dissection and rupture.

4.2.7 Pulmonary circulation

4.2.7.1 Pulmonary artery

Hypoplasia or aplasia of the pulmonary artery is often seen in complex congenital heart disease (Figure 276).

4.2.7.2 Pulmonary veins

Partial anomalous return of the pulmonary veins is seen as an isolated finding or as part of other abnormalities (Figures 280 and 313). Evidence of remote surgical repair is occasionally found (Figure 314).

4.2.8 Arteriovenous shunt defects

The ductus arteriosus is a communication between the descending aorta and the main pulmonary artery. In the fetus it physiologically bypasses pulmonary circulation. A patent ductus can be found in asymptomatic adults, in particular if the size is small (Figure 315). The fibrotic and often calcified remnant is called the ligamentum arteriosum (Figure 316).

An unusual arteriovenous (AV) malformation is shown in Figures 317 and 318.

4.2.9 Anomalous central venous return

Anomalies of the vena cava can be assessed (Figures 319 and 320).

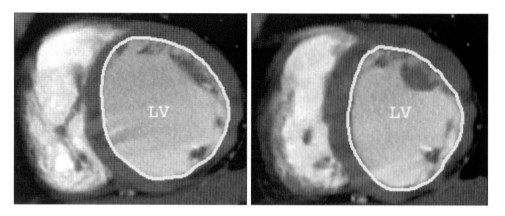

Figure 46   Left ventricular function (see also color section on p. 8)

Format: illustrated MPR

More recently, limited assessment of ventricular function has become possible with CT by combining multiple image reconstructions from different phases of the cardiac cycle into a cine-loop. The clinical role of assessing function with CT is currently being evaluated. Left ventricle (LV) measurements, including the ejection fraction (EF) from MDCT, were validated against results from cine-MRI. There was good correlation of the EF values but significant underestimation of LV volumes with MDCT.

In this figure, tracing of the left ventricular endocardial border in diastole (left panel) and systole (right panel) is shown. If performed at several levels throughout the left ventricle, the stroke volume and ejection fraction can be calculated.

CHAPTER 4.1.1, REFERENCES 57, 63, 64

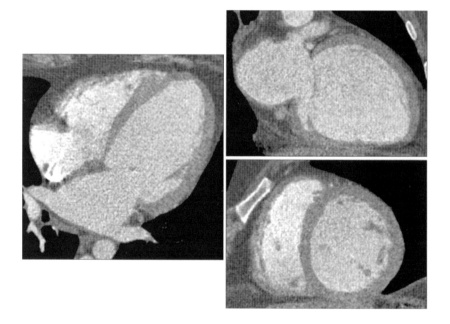

Figure 47   Dilated cardiomyopathy

Format: MPR

The typical findings in patients with dilated cardiomyopathy are ventricular dilatation with relative thinning of the myocardium. These findings can involve the left and right ventricles and are associated with ventricular dysfunction of various degrees. Because the etiology is primarily related to myocardium pathology, the coronary arteries are typically normal or only mildly diseased.

This figure shows images of a patient with suspected non-ischemic cardiomyopathy. There is moderate-to-severe left ventricular dilatation without evidence of focal scarring. There is mild-to-moderate left atrial dilatation. The right ventricle is normal. There is no evidence of thrombus within the cardiac chambers. There was no evidence of coronary artery disease.

CHAPTER 4.1.1.1, REFERENCES 65, 66

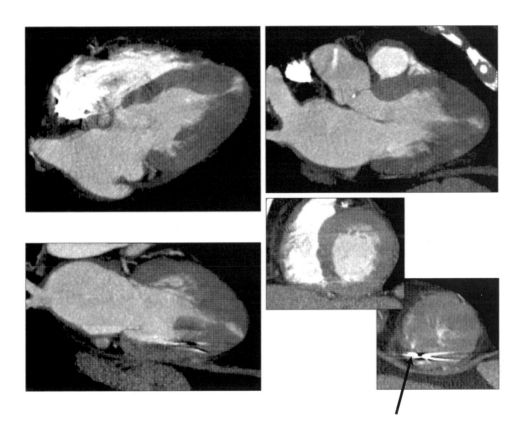

Figure 48   Apical hypertrophic cardiomyopathy (1)

Format: MIP

Hypertrophic cardiomyopathies (HCMs) are characterized by primary ventricular hypertrophy with characteristic distribution of the hypertrophic myocardium. Apical HCM (Yamaguchi) is characterized by concentric left ventricular thickening in the distal and apical segments.

The typical distribution of apical hypertrophy is shown in this and the following figure. Systolic contraction leads to obstruction of the distal left ventricular cavity. The wire of a defibrillator system (ICD) is seen ending in the right ventricle (arrow).

CHAPTER 4.1.1.1, REFERENCES 65, 67

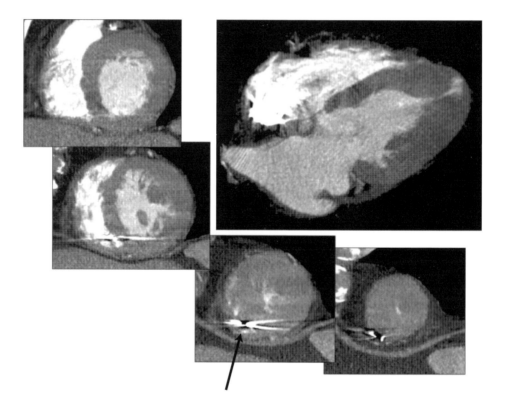

Figure 49   Apical hypertrophic cardiomyopathy (2)

Format: MIP

The findings are further illustrated in this figure. Cross-sectional short-axis images through the left ventricle show the asymmetric, distal and apical myocardial thickening. The pacer wire is seen (arrow).

CHAPTER 4.1.1.1, REFERENCES 65, 67

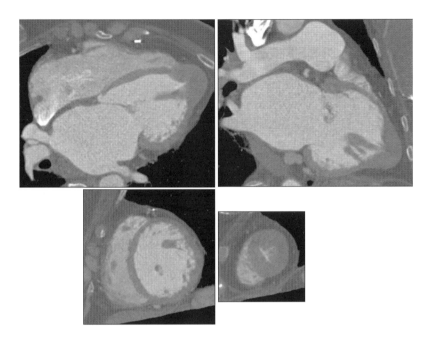

Figure 50 Atypical apical hypertrophic cardiomyopathy

Format: MPR

An atypical distribution of focal hypertrophy, limited to the left ventricular apex, is shown in this figure.

CHAPTER 4.1.1.1, REFERENCES 65, 67

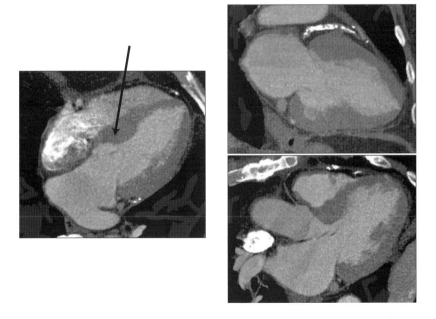

Figure 51 Hypertrophic obstructive cardiomyopathy (HOCM)

Format: MIP

The classic morphologic finding in patients with hypertrophic obstructive cardiomyopathy is asymmetric septal hypertrophy. However, functional evidence of outflow tract obstruction (typically obtained by echocardiography) is necessary for the diagnosis.

This figure shows images of a patient with hypertrophic obstructive cardiomyopathy. Asymmetric hypertrophy of the proximal interventricular septum is seen (arrow). Echocardiography demonstrated outflow tract obstruction. In addition to the myocardial findings, dense calcification of the LAD coronary artery is seen.

CHAPTER 4.1.1.1, REFERENCES 65, 67

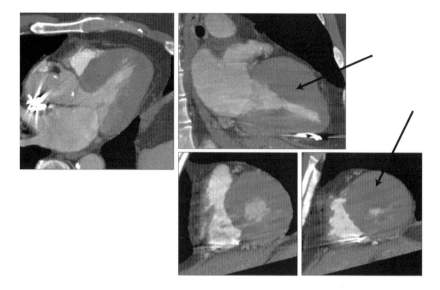

Figure 52   Hypertrophic non-obstructive cardiomyopathy (HCM)

Format: MIP

Non-obstructive hypertrophic cardiomyopathy is differentiated from HOCM by the absence of outflow tract obstruction. This figure shows images of a patient with severe diffuse left ventricular hypertrophy with focal prominence of the anterior wall (arrows) but no morphologic evidence of outflow tract obstruction. The absence of fixed or dynamic functional obstruction was confirmed by echocardiography. The pattern suggests a form of hypertrophic non-obstructive cardiomyopathy.

CHAPTER 4.1.1.1, REFERENCES 65, 67

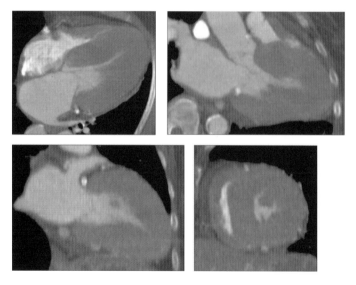

Figure 53   Cardiac amyloidosis

Format: MIP

Restrictive cardiomyopathy describes a group of disease conditions which are characterized by increased ventricular stiffness. Diagnostic hallmarks are early diastolic dysfunction, which is best assessed with echocardiography. Ventricular stiffness can be secondary to myocardial infiltration, where advanced disease stages potentially show myocardial prominence and can involve both the left and the right ventricular wall.

These findings are demonstrated in this figure, which shows severe left- and right-sided wall thickening with overall diffuse enlargement of the left ventricle. The ventricular wall has a thickness of 3.0 cm on the left and 1 cm on the right. This appearance is unusual for left ventricular hypertrophy secondary to hypertensive heart disease, and is consistent with an infiltrative process including amyloidosis or hypertrophic cardiomyopathy.

CHAPTER 4.1.1.1, REFERENCES 63, 65, 68

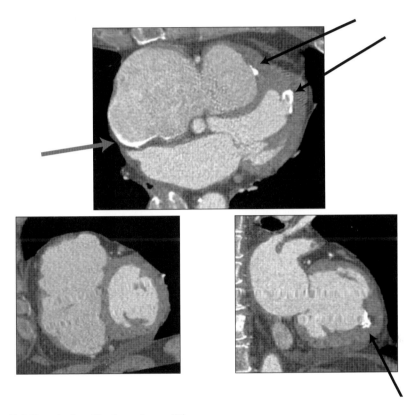

Figure 54   Endocardial fibrosis: Loeffler's endocarditis

Format: MPR

Alternatively, restriction can be caused by endocardial fibrosis. This is demonstrated in these images of a patient with a history of Loeffler's endocarditis.

There is a small pericardial effusion. There is severe enlargement of the right atrium and moderately severe enlargement of the right ventricle with a reversal of normal interventricular septal curvature. There are bulky areas of calcification in the myocardium of the right and left ventricular apices (thin arrows), with blunting of the ventricular cavities and deformity in the configuration of both ventricles due to apical scar tissue combined with dense calcification. The calcification in the right atrium is consistent with a layered, calcified thrombus (thick arrow).

CHAPTER 4.1.1.1, REFERENCES 65

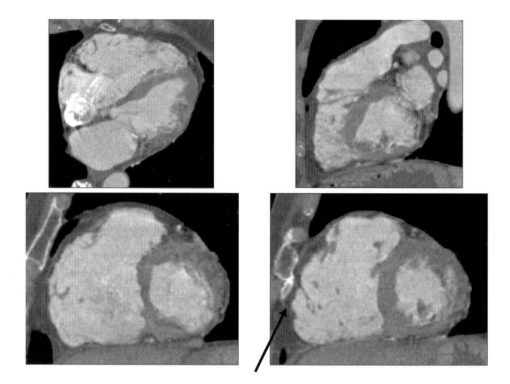

Figure 55 Arrhythmogenic right ventricular dysplasia (ARVD) (1)

Format: MPR

Arrhythmogenic right ventricular dysplasia is a clinical syndrome of life-threatening ventricular tachycardia originating from foci of a remodeled right ventricular wall. Major and minor diagnostic criteria (clinical, electrocardiographic, imaging, etc.) have been described. Major imaging criteria are global right ventricular dysfunction, global right ventricular cavity dilatation and focal right ventricular wall aneurysm formation. Minor imaging criteria are focal wall thinning with fibrous or fatty replacement of myocardium involving the right ventricular and sometimes left ventricular myocardium.

The images of this figure demonstrate major findings including moderate dilatation of the right ventricle. Further evaluation of the right ventricular wall is notable for small aneurysms of the wall (arrow) and probable fibrofatty replacement of its myocardium. Together these abnormalities are supportive of the diagnosis of ARVD.

CHAPTER 4.1.1.1, REFERENCES 69–73

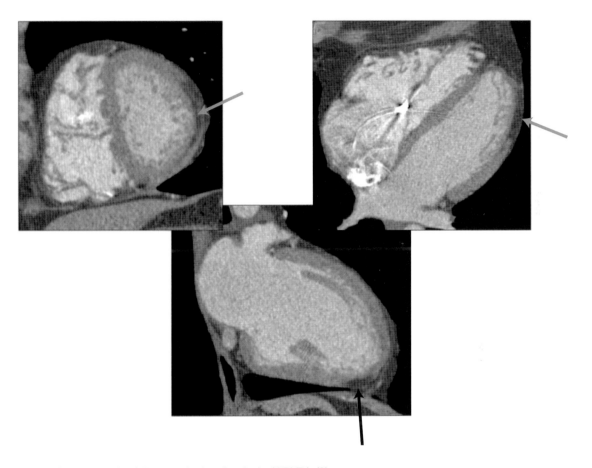

Figure 56   Arrhythmogenic right ventricular dysplasia (ARVD) (2)

Format: MPR

In this patient with ARVD there is at most mild dilatation of the right ventricle. However, there is significant fibrofatty replacement of the right ventricular myocardium, seen by the lack of differentiation between epicardial fat and right ventricular myocardium (compare with normal right ventricular wall morphology in Figure 37). Importantly, there is an area of fatty replacement of the left ventricular myocardium (arrows).

CHAPTER 4.1.1.1, REFERENCES 69–73

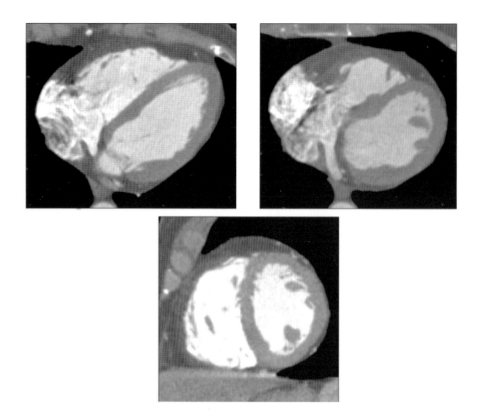

Figure 57 Arrhythmogenic right ventricular dysplasia (ARVD) (3)

Format: MIP

This figure shows evidence of pronounced fatty replacement of the right ventricular myocardium with fatty material. This is seen throughout the right ventricular outflow tract as well as the right ventricular body. Functional assessment with MRI demonstrated overall normal right ventricular size and function. However, there was regional systolic dysfunction of the anterior wall.

CHAPTER 4.1.1.1, REFERENCES 69–73

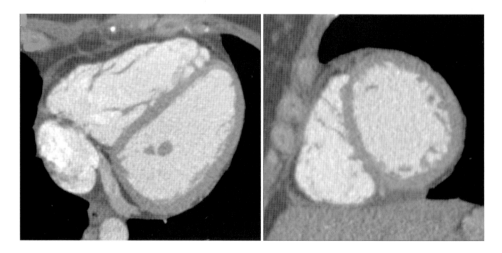

Figure 58 Arrhythmogenic right ventricular dysplasia (ARVD) (4)

Format: MPR

A more subtle case of focal wall thinning with fibrous or fatty replacement of myocardium is shown here. However, comparison with a normal right ventricular wall (Figure 37) demonstrates the different wall morphology.

CHAPTER 4.1.1.1, REFERENCES 69–73

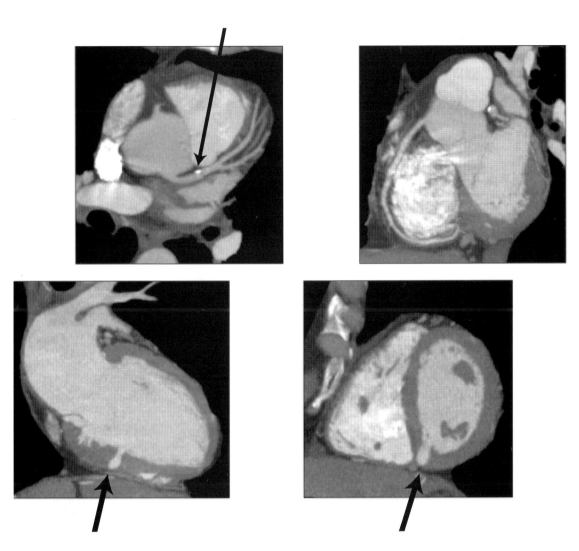

Figure 59   Left ventricular diverticulum

Format: MIP

Left ventricular diverticula are small, congenital outpouchings of the left ventricular cavity with relatively maintained wall structure. Diverticula can be differentiated from focal aneurysms by the maintained contractility on functional studies (Movies 13 and 14).

This figure shows a focal diverticulum of the left ventricular cavity (thick arrows), which extends into the inferior wall near the mid-interventricular septum. There is focal thinning of the left ventricular wall but the area is surrounded by myocardium. In the differential diagnosis an incomplete muscular ventricular sepal defect (VSD) should be considered. In contrast to post-infarct aneurysms, there is only mild coronary artery disease of the LAD (thin arrow).

CHAPTER 4.1.1.2, REFERENCES 61–63, 65

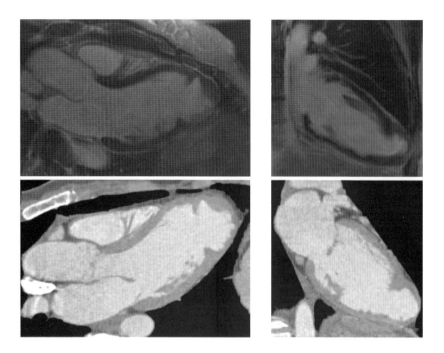

Figure 60   Left ventricular apical diverticulum

Format: MPR, MRI

This figure shows images of a patient with a left ventricular apical diverticulum. MRI and CT images are shown in the upper and lower panels, respectively. At the left ventricular apex, there is a relatively thin-walled saccular outpouching in communication with the main cavity of the left ventricle. The wall of the outpouching comprises myocardial tissue demonstrating systolic contraction on MRI (Movies 13 and 14) and measures 4.6 cm × 3.0 cm. There is no evidence of fibrosis or calcification of the wall and no thrombus within its cavity.

CHAPTER 4.1.1.2, REFERENCES 61–63, 65

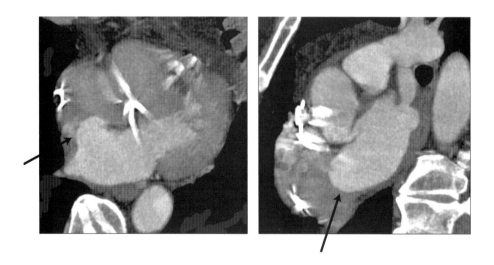

Figure 61   Atrial septal aneurysm

Format: MIP

The intra-atrial septum and fibrous part of the intraventricular septum can demonstrate aneurysmal bulging. This figure demonstrates an aneurysm of the intra-atrial septum bulging toward the right atrium (arrows) without definitive morphologic evidence of atrial septal defect (ASD). However, further assessment of shunt flow requires examination with echocardiography and MRI.

CHAPTER 4.1.1.2, REFERENCES 61–63, 65

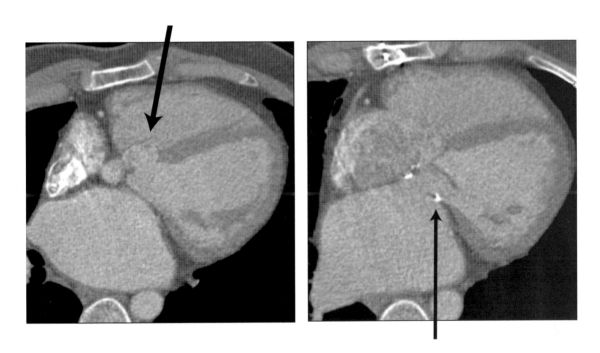

Figure 62   Ventricular septal aneurysm

Format: MPR

This figure demonstrates an aneurysm of the fibrous intraventricular septum (thick arrow) bulging toward the right ventricle without morphologic evidence of a VSD. There is evidence of mitral valve repair with a valvular ring (thin arrow).

CHAPTER 4.1.1.2, REFERENCES 61–63, 65

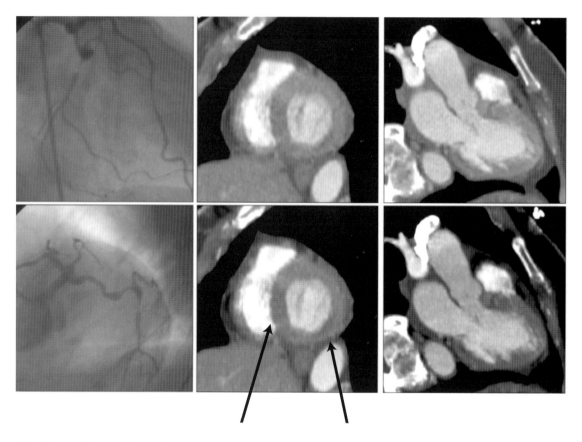

Figure 63   Myocardial perfusion defect

Format: angiogram, MPR, MIP

Animal models and occasional clinical observations describe areas of decreased contrast enhancement in hypoperfused myocardial segments.

This figure shows an example of a perfusion defect of the inferior-posterior and septal wall. The patient presented to an emergency room with back pain. There was initial concern of aortic dissection, and a CT of the chest and abdomen was performed. The posterolateral and inferoseptal regions demonstrate decreased subendocardial contrast enhancement consistent with hypoperfusion (arrows). This area is better seen on the MIP images (lower panel). On the angiogram there is diffuse, severely stenotic atherosclerotic disease of the left circumflex and left anterior descending coronary arteries.

CHAPTER 4.1.1.3, REFERENCES 74–78

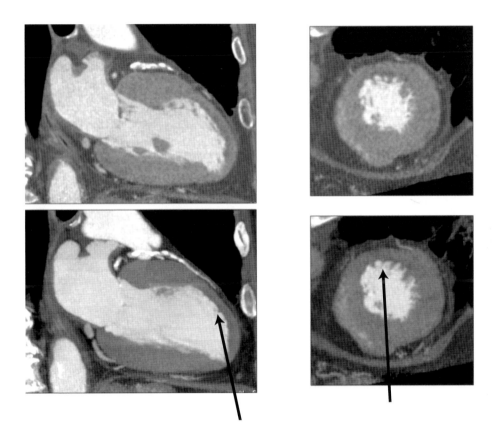

Figure 64 Chronic myocardial perfusion defect

Format: MPR, MIP

It is currently not completely understood whether areas of decreased contrast enhancement can differentiate between acute and chronic changes.

This figure shows an example of a chronic perfusion defect of the anterior wall. The patient had a remote history of myocardial infarction and had a CT performed to define aortic anatomy. The cardiac chambers are notable for mild left ventricular hypertrophy except for the mid- to apical anterior wall, corresponding to the LAD distribution, which shows myocardial thinning, consistent with previous myocardial infarction. There is a small area of decreased subendocardial contrast enhancement consistent with hypoperfusion (arrows). This area is better seen on the MIP images (lower panels). Corresponding to the area of previous infarction, the LAD has diffuse atherosclerotic changes with densely calcified lesions.

CHAPTER 4.1.1.3, REFERENCES 74–78

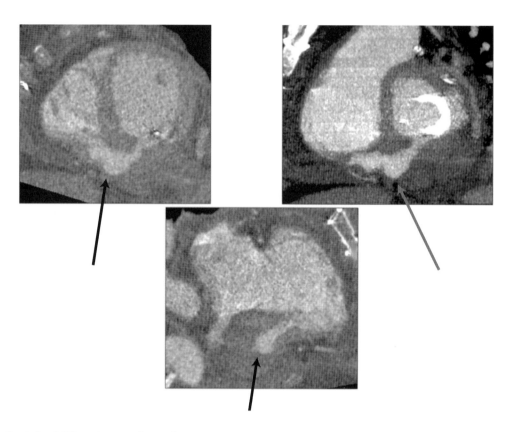

Figure 65   Contained LV rupture and pseudoaneurysm

Format: MPR, MIP

CT has an established role in the evaluation of subacute complications of acute myocardial infarction, including free wall rupture and pseudoaneurysm formation.

This figure shows short-axis (upper panels) and two-chamber (lower panel) images from a patient with an inferobasal left ventricular pseudoaneurysm after acute myocardial infarction. A partially contrast-filled pseudoaneurysm originates from the inferior aspect of the left ventricle and extends under both ventricles (arrows). There is evidence of mitral valve replacement with a bioprosthetic valve.

CHAPTER 4.1.1.3, REFERENCES 80, 81

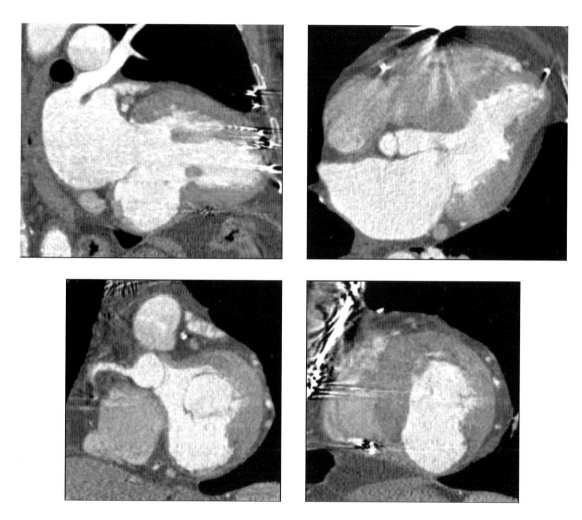

Figure 66 LV pseudoaneurysm

Format: MPR

This figure shows images from a patient with an inferobasal left ventricular pseudoaneurysm after an acute myocardial infarction. A contrast-filled pseudoaneurysm originates from the basal inferior aspect of the left ventricle and extends under the mitral valve.

CHAPTER 4.1.1.3, REFERENCES 65, 81

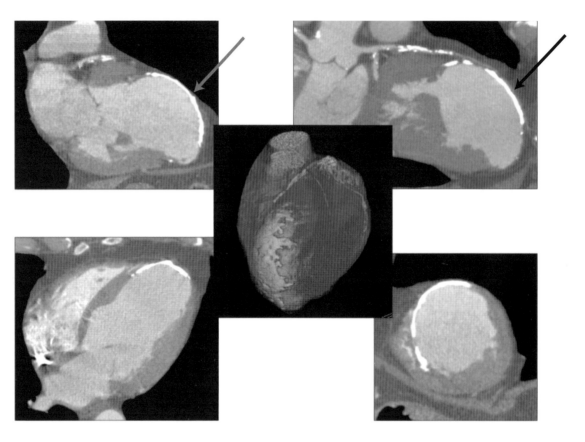

Figure 67   Calcified left ventricular aneurysm (1) (see also color section on p. 9)

Format: MPR, VRI

Areas of remote left ventricular myocardial infarction typically demonstrate ventricular wall thinning with fibrous or calcified replacement of myocardium, and aneurysm formation with or without cavitary thrombus.

This figure shows images of a patient with coronary artery disease. There is dense calcified disease of the proximal to mid-LAD, with a post-infarct aneurysm of the anterior left ventricular myocardium (arrows). There is overall moderate left ventricular dilatation. Beginning at the junction of the proximal and middle thirds of the left ventricle, there is pronounced myocardial thinning including the anterior and septal segments, with relative sparing of the anterolateral and lateral regions. The area of thinning demonstrates bulging compatible with true aneurysm formation extending to the apex. The infarcted wall is densely calcified without evidence of adherent mural thrombus.

CHAPTER 4.1.1.3, REFERENCES 65, 81

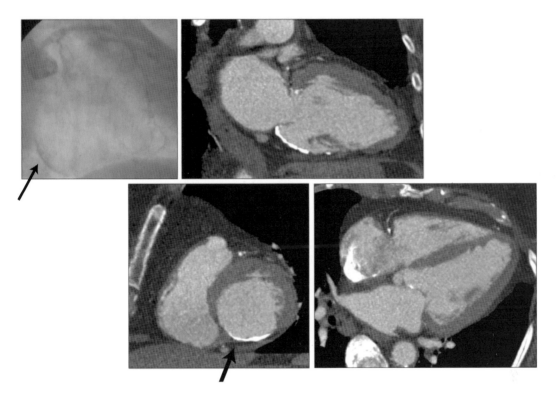

Figure 68   Calcified left ventricular aneurysm (2)

Format: MIP, angiogram

This figure shows images of a patient with known coronary artery disease. During a cardiac catheterization, an area of calcification in the inferior basal segment of the left ventricle was noted and pericardial calcification was suspected (thin arrow, left upper panel).

However, the subsequent CT demonstrated myocardial calcification consistent with a myocardial scar (thick arrow). The left ventricle is notable for myocardial thinning of the basal and mid-inferior walls. There is associated calcification of the base of the inferior wall beginning at the level of the mitral annulus. The pericardium has normal thickness without evidence of calcification. There is severe calcification of all three coronary arteries. These findings are consistent with remote myocardial infarction.

CHAPTER 4.1.1.3, REFERENCES 65, 81

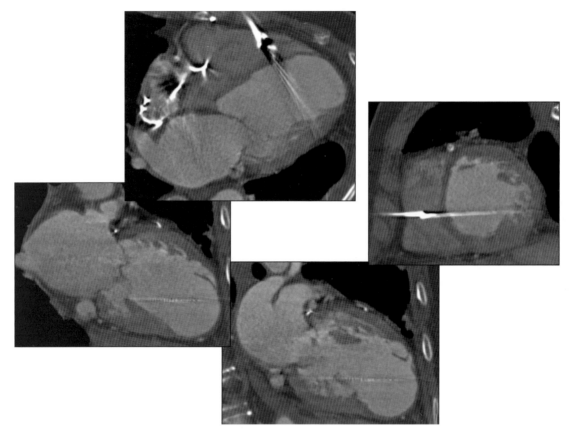

Figure 69   Ischemic cardiomyopathy: assessment of scar tissue

Format: MPR

This figure shows images of a patient with ischemic cardiomyopathy and prior coronary bypass surgery. The patient is evaluated for possible re-do open heart surgery. There is concern for ventricular geometry and areas of myocardial scar tissue. Because of an ICD/pacemaker device with leads into the right ventricle, a MRI examination could not be performed.

There are severe calcified atherosclerotic changes of the native coronary arteries. There is evidence of prior coronary bypass surgery with a patent LIMA graft to the LAD, and patent aorto-coronary grafts to the left circumflex coronary artery and a diagonal branch of the LAD. There is a stump of an aorto-coronary graft to the RCA (grafts not shown in the figure).

There is moderate left ventricular dilatation and moderate left atrial dilatation. There is thinning of the septal, anteroseptal and inferoseptal myocardium in the mid- and distal segments, consistent with a myocardial scar. There is thinning and bulging of the left ventricular apex, consistent with an aneurysm. There is no evidence of thrombus. The remaining segments of the myocardium have normal thickness.

The right ventricle has normal dimensions.

CHAPTER 4.1.1.3, REFERENCES 65, 81

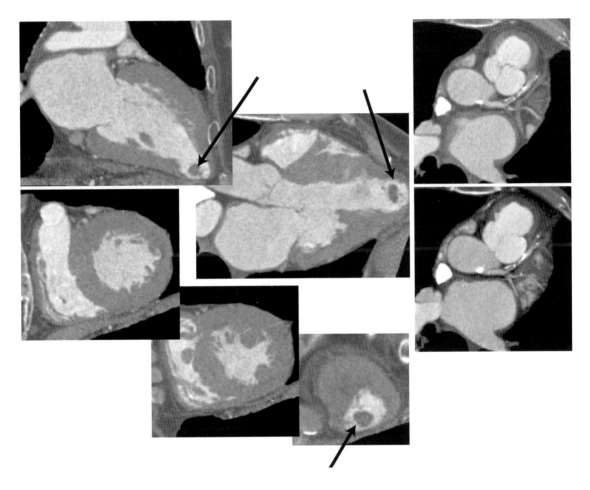

Figure 70   Small apical left ventricular aneurysm

Format: MPR, MIP

This figure shows a small left ventricular apical aneurysm containing a thrombus (arrows). Significant accumulation of mixed (calcified and non-calcified) plaque and luminal narrowing is seen in the mid-LAD coronary artery (right panels).

CHAPTER 4.1.1.3, REFERENCES 65, 81

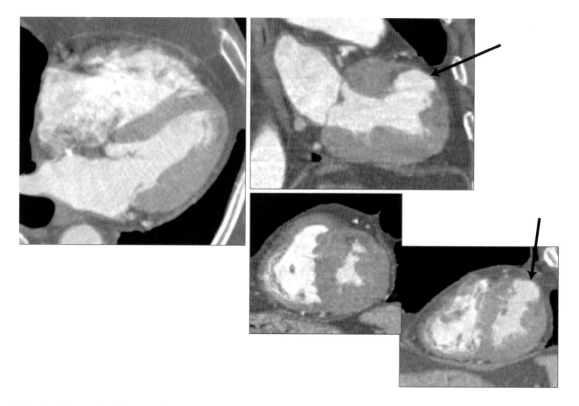

Figure 71   Small anterior left ventricular aneurysm

Format: MPR

This figure shows a small focal aneurysm of the anterior left ventricular wall. There is severe concentric left ventricular hypertrophy, with the exception of the anterior wall. In the mid-third is focal transmural scar formation (arrows). This area of remote infarction appears as an area of excavation within the thickened muscle, creating a saccular extension of the LV cavity. The area corresponded to a subtotally or totally occluded second diagonal branch of the LAD. There is no evidence of intracavitary thrombus in the infarct zone. An MRI study demonstrated focal akinesis but no diastolic bulging. Overall LV ejection fraction was 55%.

CHAPTER 4.1.1.3, REFERENCES 65, 81

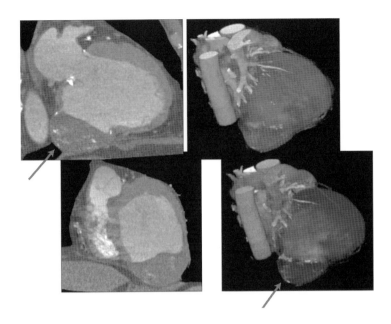

Figure 72   Large, thrombosed inferior left ventricular pseudoaneurysm

Format: MIP, VRI

This figure shows a large, thrombosed saccular pseudoaneurysm of the left ventricle, which measures 7.4 × 7.2 × 4.1 cm (arrows). There is global, severe left ventricular dilatation. Involving the inferior and posterior regions of the proximal half of the left ventricle is a saccular-appearing outpouching, which is filled with partially calcified thrombus.

There is significant coronary atherosclerosis of all three coronary arteries, with severe disease of the dominant RCA corresponding to the location of the aneurysm.

CHAPTER 4.1.1.3, REFERENCES 65, 81

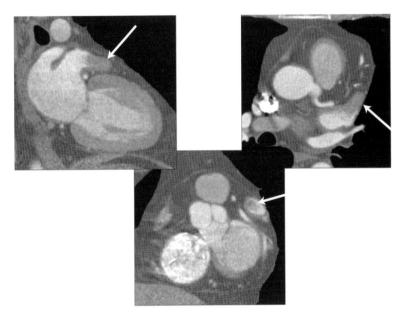

Figure 73   Left atrial appendage clot (1)

Format: MPR

Left atrial appendage (LAA) clot is common and frequently associated with atrial fibrillation. It appears as a filling defect in the appendage. However, slow flow in the left atrial appendage as described by transesophageal echocardiography may appear as an LAA filling defect on CT. LAA filling may also depend on contrast timing.

This figure shows a large filling defect in the left atrial appendage (arrow), consistent with a clot.

CHAPTER 4.1.1.4, REFERENCES 65, 82, 83

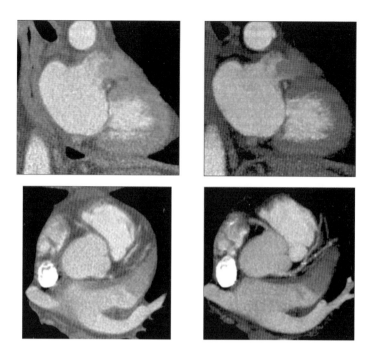

Figure 74 Left atrial appendage clot (2)

Format: MPR, MIP

Another example of a filling defect in the left atrial appendage is shown in these MPR (left panels) and MIP images (right panels).

CHAPTER 4.1.1.4, REFERENCES 65, 82, 83

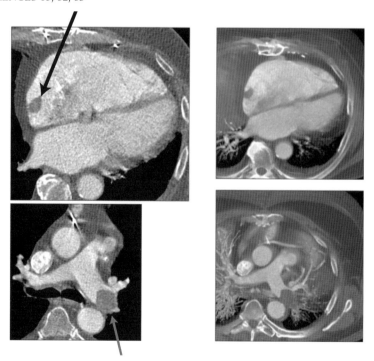

Figure 75 Right atrial thrombus

Format: MPR, VRI

Right atrial thrombus is less common, and underlying abnormalities of coagulation are often suspected. In this figure, images of a patient with pulmonary embolism (thin arrow) and right atrial thrombus (thick arrow) are shown.

CHAPTER 4.1.1.4, REFERENCES 65

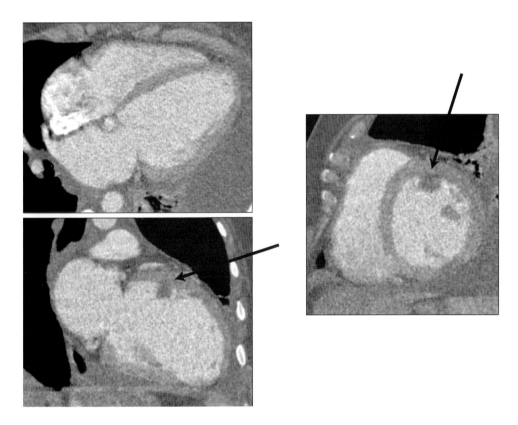

Figure 76 Left ventricular thrombus

Format: MPR

Although left ventricular thrombus is often associated with post-infarct aneurysms (Figure 70), occasional left ventricular clot without underlying LV dysfunction is found (arrows).

CHAPTER 4.1.1.4, REFERENCES 65

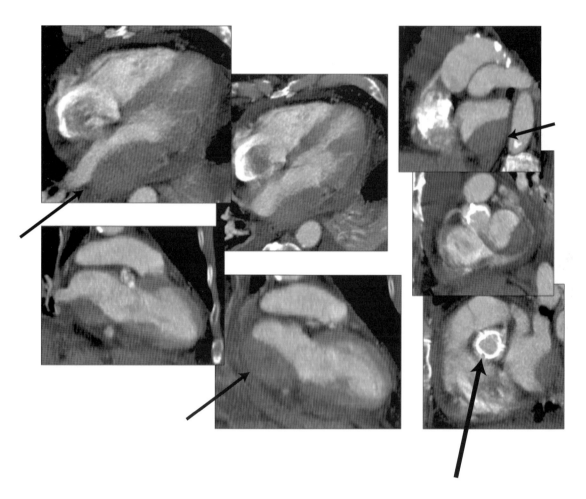

Figure 77 Postoperative left atrial wall hematoma (1.1)

Format: MIP

An unusual finding is atrial or ventricular wall hematoma after open heart surgery. This figure shows images of a patient who had recent aortic valve replacement with a Carpentier–Edwards pericardial valve and an aorto-coronary bypass graft to the right coronary artery.

The CT scan performed 5 days after surgery demonstrates a mass in the floor of the left atrium (thin arrows). The mass appears to be within the left atrial wall, with the coronary sinus draped around it. The pulmonary veins and coronary sinus are not compressed. There is a small pericardial effusion, and the aortic valve prosthesis is seen (thick arrow). The findings are consistent with a wall hematoma.

CHAPTER 4.1.1.4, REFERENCES 65

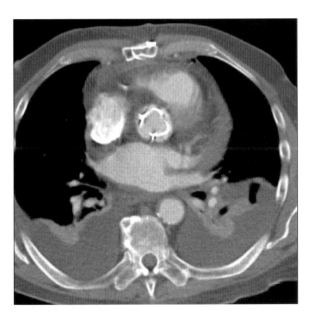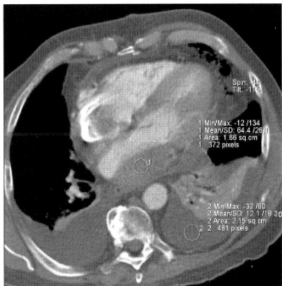

Figure 78   Postoperative left atrial wall hematoma (1.2)

Format: MPR

In this image of the same patient as in Figure 77, axial images show the suspected left atrial wall hematoma and a pleural effusion. The Hounsfield unit measurements of the atrial wall (mean 64.4) is consistent with a hematoma.

CHAPTER 4.1.1.4, REFERENCES 65

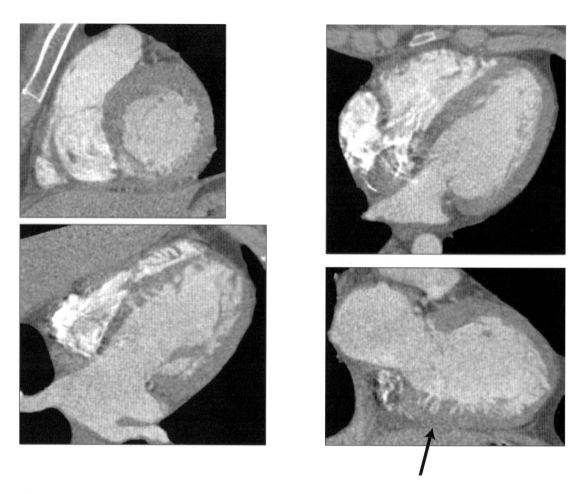

Figure 79   Left ventricular non-compaction (1)

Format: MPR

Left ventricular non-compaction describes an incidental finding of prominent left ventricular trabeculation, related to embryonic wall development.

In this figure, prominent trabeculations are obvious in the inferior and lateral walls of the left ventricle (arrow).

CHAPTER 4.1.1.5, REFERENCES 84, 85

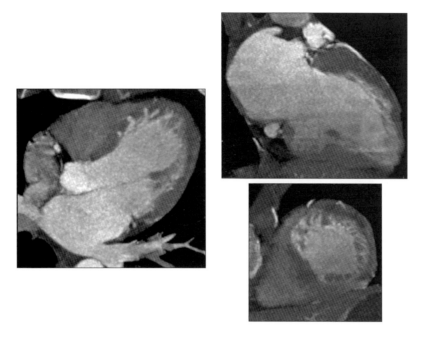

Figure 80 Left ventricular non-compaction (2.1)

Format: MPR

In this figure, images of a young patient with a history of syncope and an abnormal stress test (deep horizontal inferior ST depression and decrease in ejection fraction) are shown. The left ventricle has normal dimensions. There are pronounced trabeculations of mid- and distal anterior and inferior walls. A cardiac MRI (Movies 20–22) showed normal rest left ventricular function and no evidence of a scar. The findings are consistent with left ventricular non-compaction.

CHAPTER 4.1.1.5, REFERENCES 84, 85

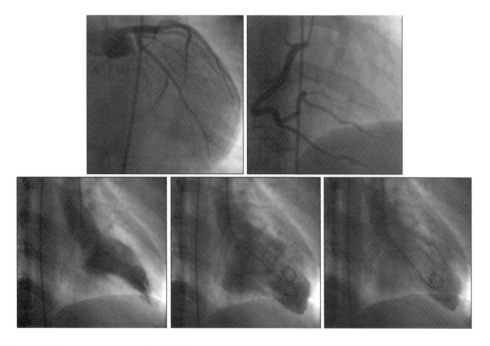

Figure 81 Left ventricular non-compaction (2.2)

Format: MPR

The corresponding angiographic images confirm the areas of trabeculation. There is no evidence of stenotic disease of the epicardial coronary arteries.

CHAPTER 4.1.1.5, REFERENCES 84, 85

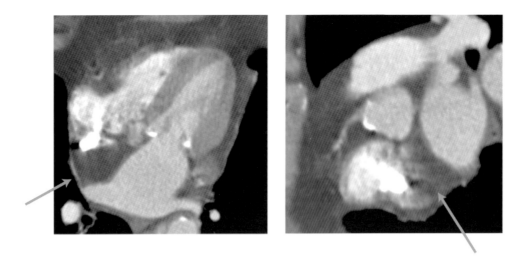

Figure 82   Lipomatous hypertrophy of the left atrial septum

Format: MPR

Lipomatous hypertrophy describes prominent fatty infiltration of the intra-atrial septum (arrows).

CHAPTER 4.1.1.5, REFERENCES 86, 87

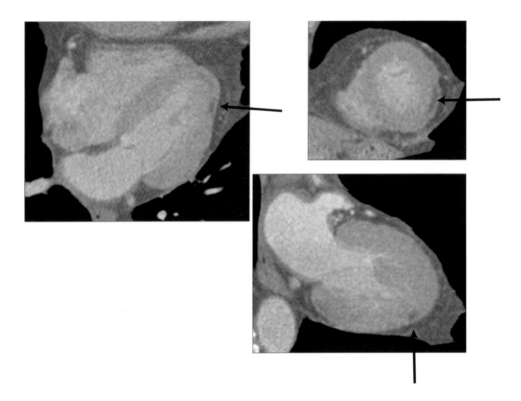

Figure 83   Myocardial scar secondary to myocarditis

Format: MPR

An unusual finding is a myocardial scar secondary to myocarditis. In contrast to scar related to coronary artery disease (CAD), the distribution of the scar tissue does not follow vascular territories and is often more focal.

These characteristics are demonstrated in this figure, showing a focal area of hypoenhancement in the inferolateral wall of the left ventricle (arrows). The CT did not show evidence of CAD.

CHAPTER 4.1.1.5, REFERENCES 65, 88

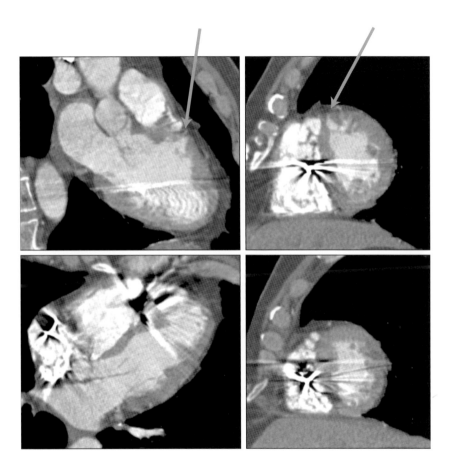

Figure 84   Cardiac sarcoidosis?

Format: MPR

Focal scar tissue not following vascular territories is also seen in cardiac sarcoidosis. This figure shows images of a patient with a history of sarcoidosis who presented with recurrent ventricular tachycardia.

Pacemaker/ICD leads extend into the right atrium and right ventricle. There is an area of focal myocardial thinning of the anteroseptal left ventricular wall in a non-vascular distribution (arrows). These findings are consistent with cardiac sarcoidosis but are not diagnostic.

CHAPTER 4.1.1.5, REFERENCES 65

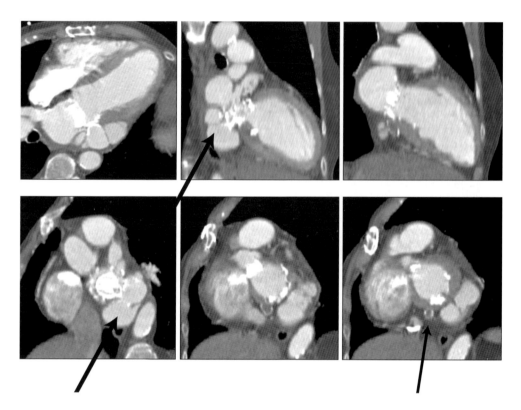

Figure 85   Postoperative pseudoaneurysm of left ventricle originating at mitral annulus

Format: MPR

This figure shows images of a patient with a remote history of aortic and mitral valve replacement. There is evidence of aortic valve and mitral valve replacement with mechanical valves. Originating from the inferolateral and lateral aspect of the mitral annulus is a contrast-filled space measuring 6.5 × 4.8 cm (thick arrows). It extends along the lateral wall of the left atrium and basal segments of the left ventricle. Its borders are partially calcified. It communicates at the level of the mitral valve prosthesis with the left ventricle. In addition, there is a small outpouching originating from the inferior aspect of the mitral annulus (thin arrow), which is thrombosed and has calcification of the wall. It measures 1.0 × 1.9 cm. These findings are consistent with postoperative pseudoaneurysms.

CHAPTER 4.1.1.5, REFERENCES 65

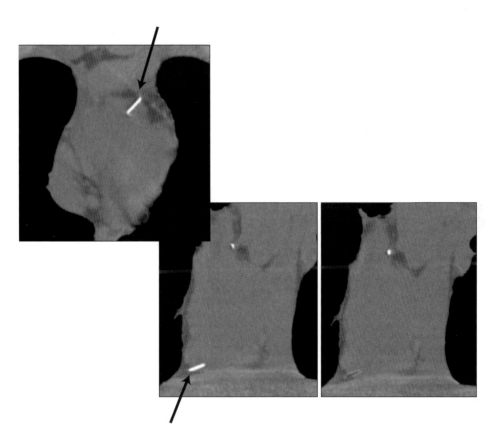

Figure 86 Needle fragment in right ventricular myocardium

Format: MPR

An anecdotal finding is shown in this figure of a patient with a history of intravenous drug abuse. The non-contrast-enhanced images show a fragment of an injection needle in the right ventricular apex (arrows), which appears to be embedded within the myocardial wall.

CHAPTER 4.1.1.5, REFERENCES 65

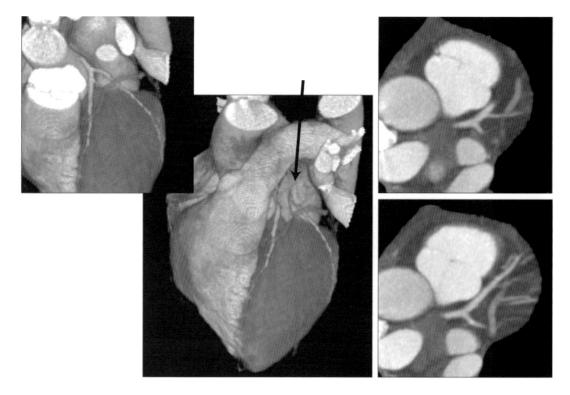

Figure 87   Normal coronary anatomy (1.1)

Format: VRI, MPR

Modern CT imaging allows a comprehensive assessment of the coronary anatomy. This figure shows findings of a normal left coronary artery. The central panel shows a volume-rendered image of the heart with the left anterior descending and left circumflex coronary arteries emerging under the left atrial appendage (arrow). The panel in the left upper corner demonstrates the left main origin of the aorta and the bifurcation below the left atrial appendage. The great cardiac vein, which is faintly enhanced, is seen crossing over the LAD and LCX. The two panels on the right show MPR images of the distal LM and proximal LAD and LCX, including the first diagonal branch of the LAD. The lumen is patent and no plaque accumulation is seen in the vessel wall.

CHAPTER 4.1.2, REFERENCES 27, 89–92

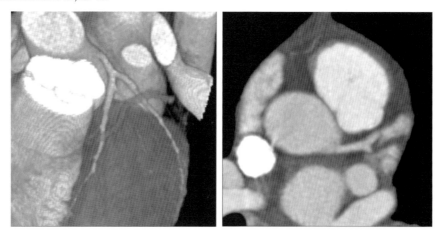

Figure 88   Normal coronary anatomy (1.2)

Format: VRI, MPR

This figure shows an enlarged image of the left main coronary artery. The VRI in the left panel shows the origin of the LM of the aorta. The MPR image on the right shows the proximal LM segment. There is no luminal stenosis or plaque accumulation.

CHAPTER 4.1.2, REFERENCES 27, 89–92

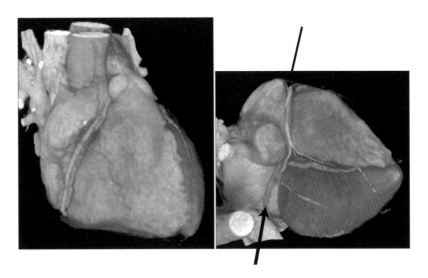

Figure 89   Normal coronary anatomy (1.3)

Format: VRI

The VRI images in this figure show the course of the right coronary artery (RCA) (thin arrow). The distal branch, the posterior descending coronary artery, at the inferior surface of the heart is shown. The coronary sinus is also visible and must be differentiated from the arterial system (thick arrow).

CHAPTER 4.1.2, REFERENCES 27, 89–92

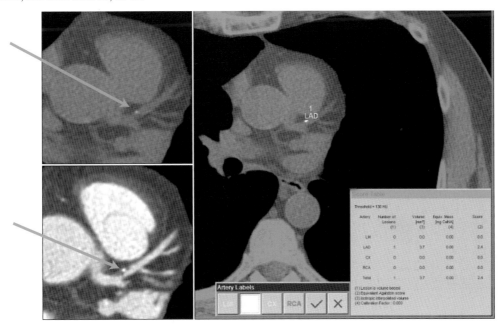

Figure 90   Calcium scoring (see also color section on p. 9)

Format: MPR

The identification of coronary arterial calcification is a reliable sign of chronic atherosclerotic changes. Advanced, stenotic lesions causing chronic, stable angina pectoris often demonstrate dense calcifications. In contrast, high-risk culprit lesions causing acute coronary events are frequently non-calcified or show microcalcification on histology. CT examinations performed without contrast administration are very sensitive in detecting and quantifying coronary arterial calcification.

The right panel shows a non-contrast-enhanced 'calcium scoring' image of a patient with a small calcification in the proximal left anterior descending coronary artery (LAD). The calcification is identified by its Hounsfield value above 130 and is color-coded. Comparison of the non-contrast-enhanced image (left upper panel) and contrast-enhanced image (left lower panel) shows that the calcified plaque is part of a larger non-calcified plaque (arrows).

CHAPTER 4.1.2.1, REFERENCES 98–123

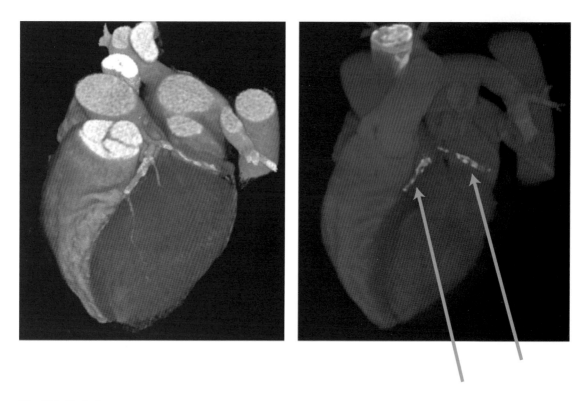

Figure 91   Calcified plaque

Format: VRI

In these volume-rendered images of a contrast-enhanced CT acquisition, changing the opacity of the data set demonstrates the location of the coronary wall calcification. There is significant calcified plaque burden of the proximal left anterior descending (LAD) and left circumflex (LCX) coronary arteries (arrows).

CHAPTER 4.1.2.1, REFERENCES 98–123

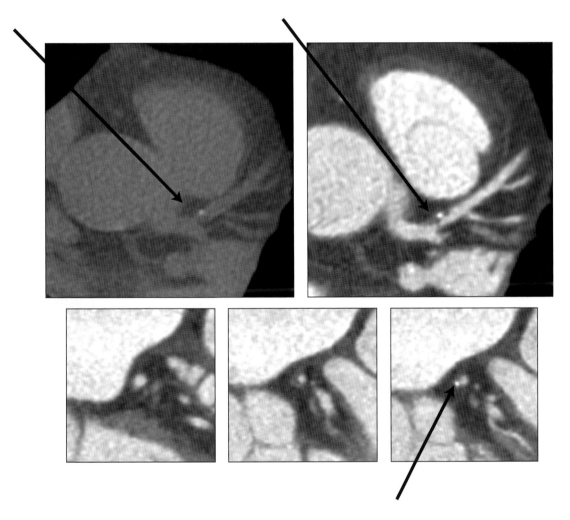

Figure 92   Calcified and non-calcified plaque (1)

Format: MPR (64-slice)

Coronary calcium scores correlate with the total atherosclerotic plaque burden (calcified and non-calcified plaque). However, the absolute burden is significantly underestimated. Despite the predictive value of the overall EBCT calcium score for future coronary events, the site of calcification does not localize the future event, which may be related to non-calcified plaque.

These limitations are demonstrated by the comparison of a non contrast-enhanced image (left upper panel) and contrast-enhanced images (right upper panel and lower panels), which demonstrates that the calcified plaque is only part of a larger non-calcified plaque (arrows).

CHAPTER 4.1.2.1, REFERENCES 93–97, 114, 115

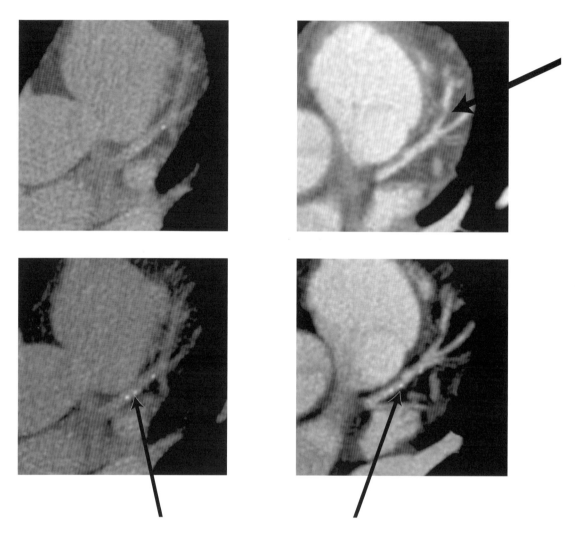

Figure 93   Calcified and non-calcified plaque (2)

Format: MPR

Only contrast-enhanced CT scans allow differentiation of lumen and vessel wall and subsequently the identification of both calcified and non-calcified plaque.

This is demonstrated in the comparison of contrast-enhanced (right panels) and non-contrast-enhanced (left panels) images of the same patient. There is calcified atherosclerotic plaque in the proximal LAD, which is not associated with luminal stenosis (thin arrows). However, there is an additional non-calcified lesion in the mid-LAD, which is associated with significant luminal stenosis (thick arrow).

CHAPTER 4.1.2.1, REFERENCES 93–97, 114, 115

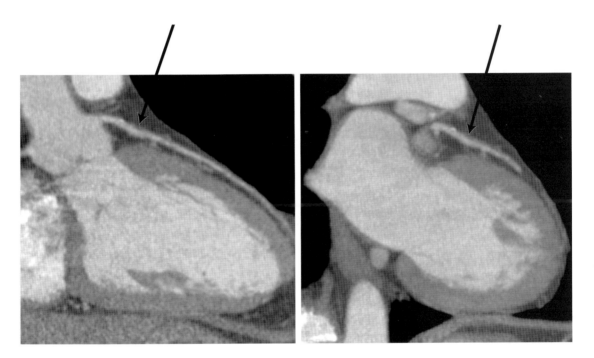

Figure 94   Coronary plaque without significant luminal stenosis

Format: curved MPR, MPR

Similar to the experience with intravascular ultrasound imaging (IVUS), emerging studies demonstrate the frequent presence of plaque burden in angiographically normal segments.

This image shows curved MPR (left panel) and straight MPR (right panel) images of a left anterior descending coronary artery (LAD) with plaque in the proximal segment (arrows). Because of expansion of the vessel area (expansive remodeling) there is no significant luminal stenosis.

CHAPTER 4.1.2.1, REFERENCES 124–128, 134–136

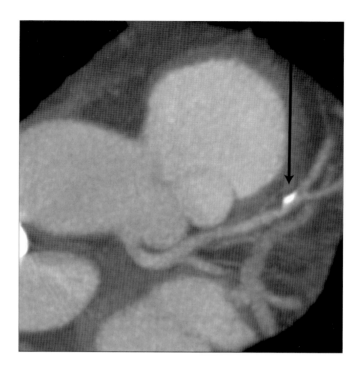

Figure 95   Calcified plaque with non-significant luminal stenosis

Format: MPR

Another example of calcified plaque in the proximal LAD without significant luminal stenosis is shown in this figure (arrow).

CHAPTER 4.1.2.1, REFERENCES 124–128, 134–136

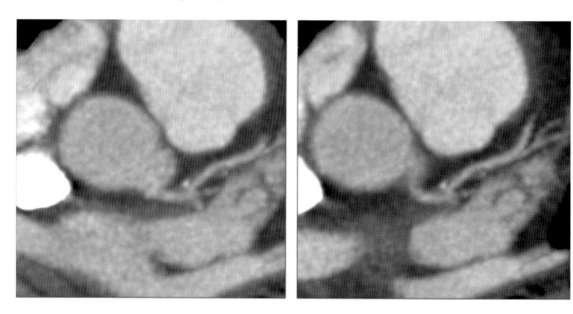

Figure 96   Arterial remodeling (1)

Format: MPR

Recent MDCT studies also describe the association of plaque accumulation with outward expansion of the vessel wall (expansive remodeling), maintaining luminal dimension.

This figure shows a mixed plaque in the left main coronary artery and non-calcified plaque in the proximal left descending coronary artery. Because of expansion of the vessel area (expansive arterial remodeling) there is no significant luminal stenosis.

CHAPTER 4.1.2.1, REFERENCES 124–128, 134–136

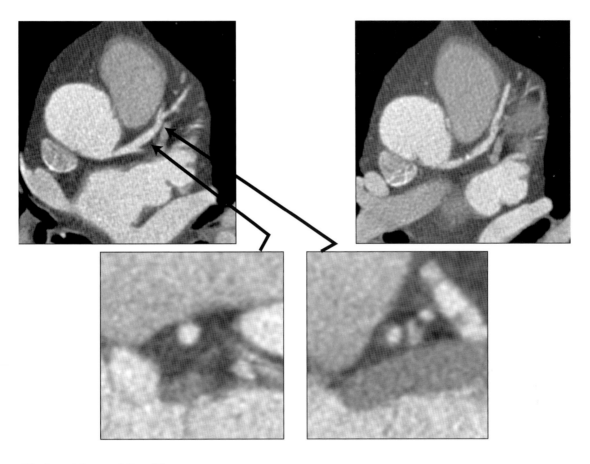

Figure 97   Arterial remodeling (2)

Format: MPR

Expansive remodeling is also demonstrated in these images of a patient who underwent preoperative evaluation of the coronary arteries prior to planned repair of an aortic dissection.

There is mild, non-calcified plaque accumulation in the left main coronary artery and proximal LAD without significant stenosis. The cross-sectional images of the proximal reference site (left lower panel) and lesion site (right lower panel) show that significant plaque accumulation is associated with mild stenosis because of expansion of the vessel area (expansive remodeling).

CHAPTER 4.1.2.1, REFERENCES 124–128, 134–136

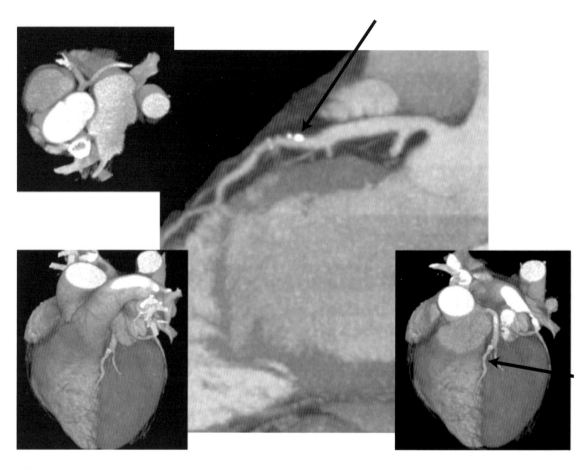

Figure 98   Mild luminal stenosis

Format: curved MPR, VRI

This figure shows images from a patient with moderate calcified disease of the LAD. The center panel shows a curved MPR image of the LAD with plaque in the proximal segments. The volume-rendered images show different views of the diseased segment. The left upper panel shows an image of the left main coronary artery, corresponding to an angiographic 'spider' view.

The 'blooming' effect of coronary calcification can result in potential overestimation of luminal stenosis, and can cause difficulties in assessing adjacent non-calcified plaque structures (arrows).

CHAPTER 4.1.2.2, REFERENCES 142–153

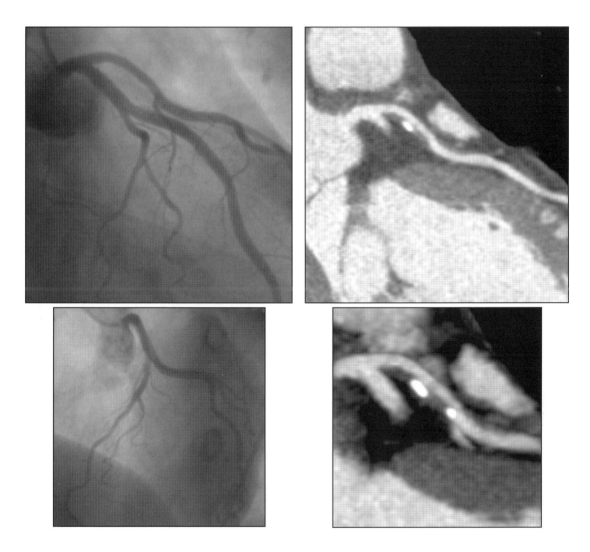

Figure 99   Moderate LAD lesion

Format: angiogram, MPR

This figure shows images from a patient with atypical chest pain. There is mixed plaque in the proximal LAD with mild angiographic stenosis, but about 50% cross-sectional narrowing in the diseased segment.
The corresponding angiogram confirms mild non-obstructive luminal stenosis.

CHAPTER 4.1.2.2, REFERENCES 142–153

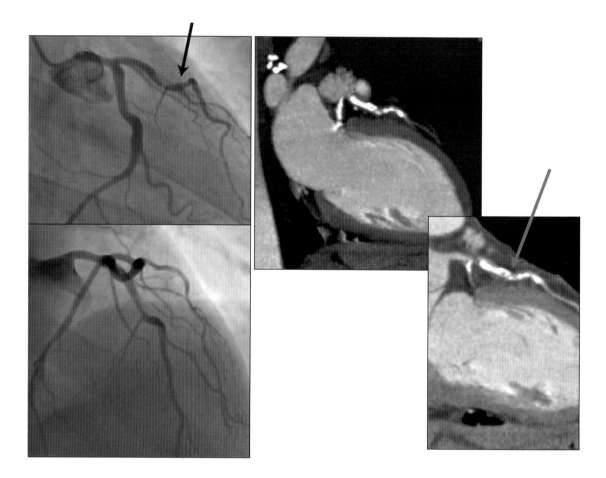

Figure 100   Moderate luminal stenosis with dense calcification

Format: angiogram, MPR, MIP

This figure shows angiographic images from a patient with moderate calcified disease of the LAD (arrow, left panels). There is significant calcified atherosclerotic plaque accumulation, which does not allow reliable assessment with CT (right panels). The arrow in the right panel shows the position corresponding to the arrow in the left panel.

CHAPTER 4.1.2.2, REFERENCES 142–153

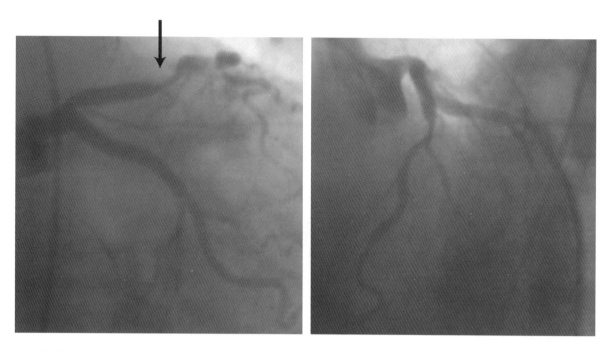

Figure 101   Significant luminal stenosis (1.1)

Format: angiogram

The following figures (101–104) compare angiographic and CT images of a significant lesion in the left anterior descending coronary artery (LAD). The angiographic images demonstrate a highly stenotic lesion of the proximal LAD with smooth borders and significant stenosis (arrow).

CHAPTER 4.1.2.2, REFERENCES 142–153

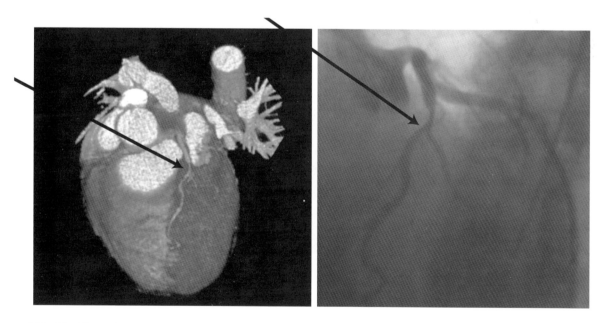

Figure 102   Significant luminal stenosis (1.2)

Format: angiogram, VRI

This figure shows a comparison between the angiogram (right panel) and a volume-rendered CT image (left panel). Both images show significant stenosis of the proximal LAD (arrows).

CHAPTER 4.1.2.2, REFERENCES 142–153

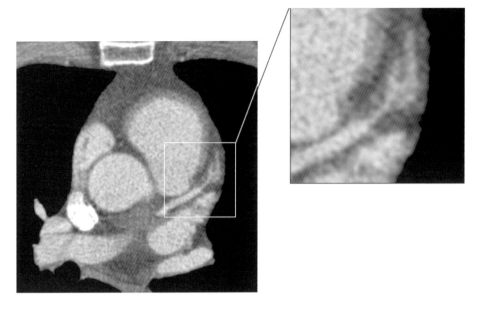

Figure 103   Significant luminal stenosis (1.3)

Format: MPR

This corresponding MPR image of the proximal LAD segment demonstrates the focal accumulation of non-calcified plaque causing luminal stenosis.

CHAPTER 4.1.2.2, REFERENCES 142–153

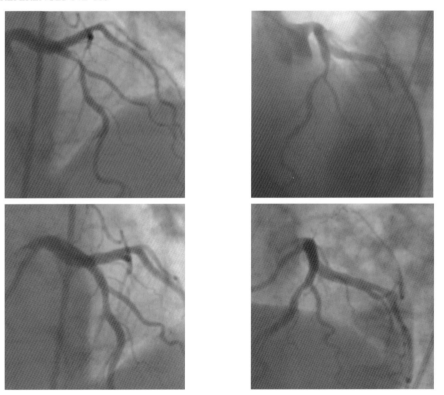

Figure 104   Significant luminal stenosis (1.4)

Format: angiogram

The patient underwent percutaneous coronary intervention. This figure shows the pre- and post-interventional angiographic images in the upper and lower panels, respectively.

CHAPTER 4.1.2.2, REFERENCES 142–153

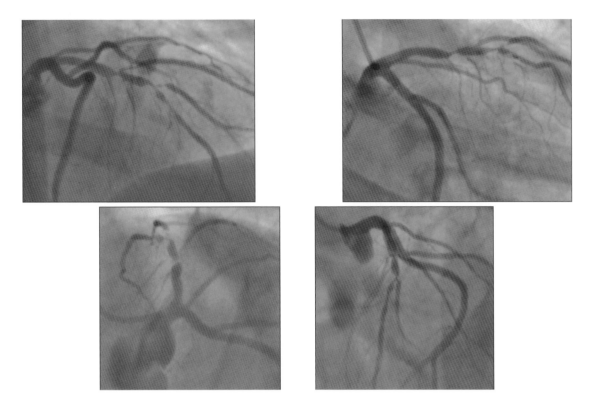

Figure 105   Significant luminal stenosis (2.1)

Format: angiogram

The strengths and limitations of non-invasive CT angiography (CTA) are demonstrated in the next figures (105–109). This figure shows angiographic images from a patient with significant luminal stenoses of the left anterior descending coronary artery (LAD).

CHAPTER 4.1.2.2, REFERENCES 142–153

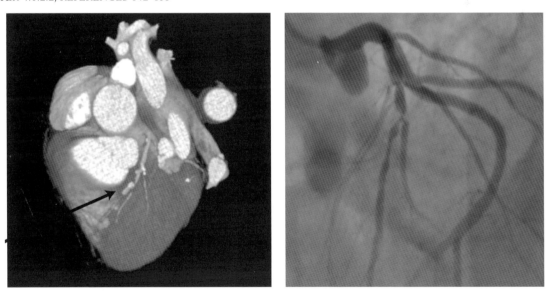

Figure 106   Significant luminal stenosis (2.2)

Format: angiogram, VRI

This figure compares an angiographic and a volume-rendered CT image. The CT shows the presence of calcified plaque in the vessel wall at the lesion site (arrow).

CHAPTER 4.1.2.2, REFERENCES 142–153

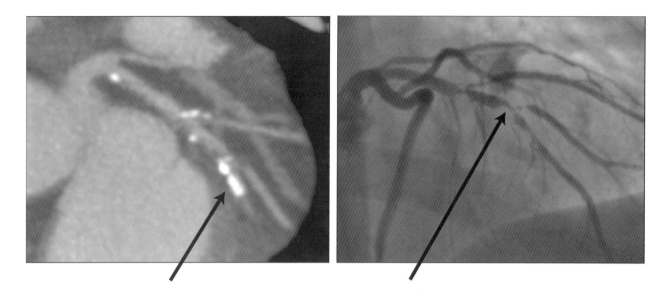

Figure 107   Significant luminal stenosis (2.3)

Format: angiogram, MPR

The dense calcification of the plaque at the lesion site is clearly shown on the MPR image (arrow). In contrast, the angiogram provides superior imaging of the luminal stenosis (arrow).

CHAPTER 4.1.2.2, REFERENCES 142–153

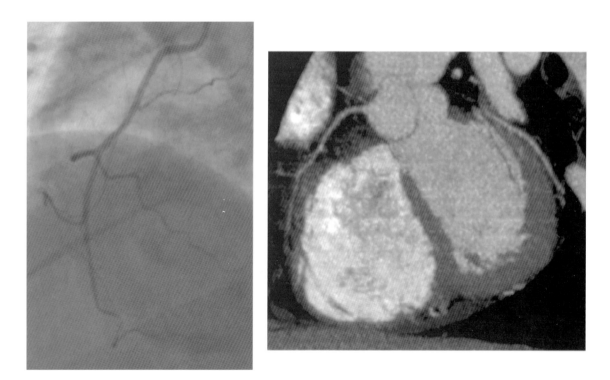

Figure 108   Significant luminal stenosis (2.4)

Format: angiogram, MIP

This figure shows a comparison between an angiographic image and a maximum intensity projection (MIP) CT image of the small, non-dominant RCA in the same patient. No significant disease is seen. Assessment of the distal segments is limited because of their small size.

CHAPTER 4.1.2.2, REFERENCES 142–153

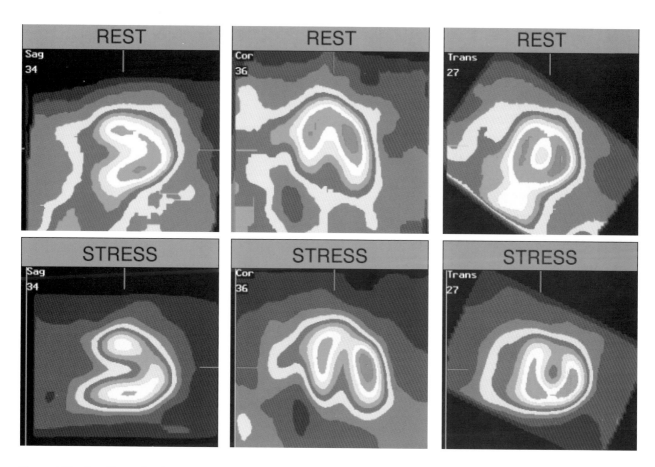

Figure 109 Significant luminal stenosis (2.5) (see also color section on p. 10)

Format: Scintigraphy

This figure shows corresponding images of the nuclear stress test. Apical ischemia, corresponding to the LAD lesions, is documented.

CHAPTER 4.1.2.2, REFERENCES 142–153

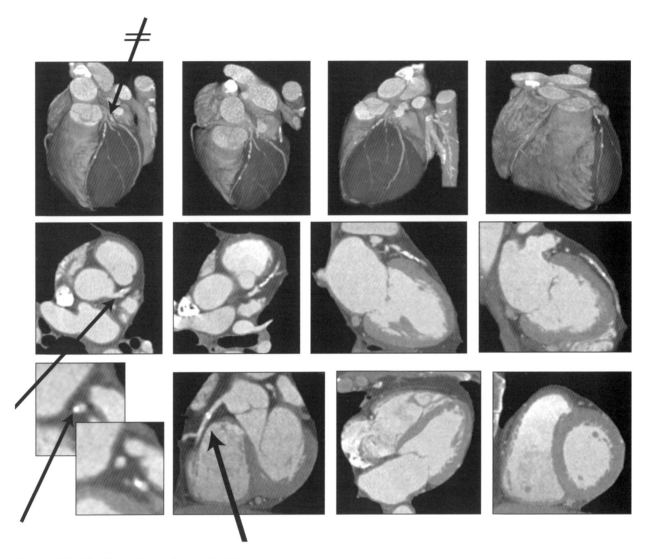

Figure 110 Significant luminal stenosis (3)

Format: MPR, VRI (64-slice scanner)

This figure shows images of a patient with known advanced obstructive coronary artery disease (CAD). Previous catheterization more than 5 years ago revealed a totally occluded proximal left anterior descending coronary artery (LAD) with filling of the distal LAD from collaterals from the right coronary artery. The patient presented with exertional chest pain and a positive positron emission tomography (PET) scan showing mild apical ischemia.

The CT scan shows a normal-size left ventricle without evidence of myocardial ischemic damage (lower right panels). There is a partially calcified atherosclerotic plaque in the ostial LAD, which causes luminal stenosis (thin arrows, left lower panels). There is dense calcification without demonstration of contrast in the proximal LAD, probably corresponding to the area of known occlusion. More distally, there are additional calcified atherosclerotic lesions.

Importantly, there is a densely calcified atherosclerotic lesion in the proximal right coronary artery (thick arrow). Although percentage stenosis cannot be assessed with CT because of the calcium 'blooming' artifact, this lesion appears to be significant. There is another densely calcified lesion of the proximal left circumflex coronary artery (crossed arrow, left upper panel).

If hemodynamically significant, the lesions in the RCA and LCX could compromise collateral flow to the distal LAD.

CHAPTER 4.1.2.2, REFERENCES 142–153

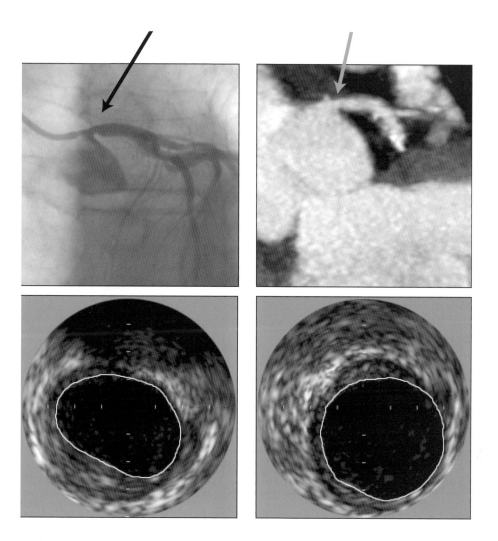

Figure 111 Left main disease

Format: angiogram, IVUS, MIP

CT may provide complementary information for subgroups of significant lesions, including assessment of unclear left main anatomy.

This figure shows images of a patient with suspected atherosclerotic disease of the left main coronary artery. The cardiac CT (right upper panel) shows ostial narrowing with suspected atherosclerotic plaque accumulation (arrow). The cardiac catheterization (left upper panel) confirmed ostial stenosis of the left main coronary artery (arrow). IVUS was performed and showed ostial atherosclerotic plaque with 30% cross-sectional narrowing (lower panels; left: ostium, right: reference site).

CHAPTER 4.1.2, REFERENCES 27, 90, 91

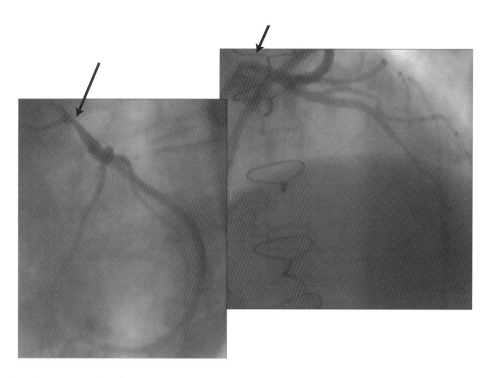

Figure 112 Left main compression (1.1)

Format: angiogram

CT may provide complementary information for subgroups of significant lesions, including assessment of unclear left main anatomy.

The following figures (112–115) show images of a patient with suspected non-atherosclerotic, external compression of the left main coronary artery. The patient has a remote history of VSD repair and presented with shortness of breath. A cardiac catheterization showed ostial stenosis of the left main coronary artery (arrows).

CHAPTER 4.1.2.2, REFERENCES 27, 90, 91

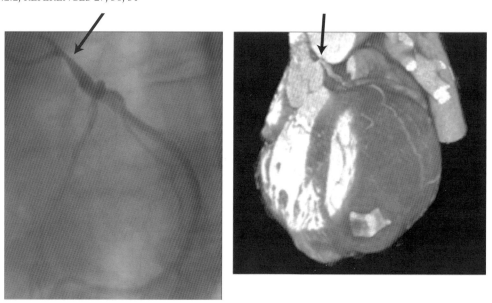

Figure 113 Left main compression (1.2)

Format: angiogram, VRI

This figure shows a comparison between angiographic and volume-rendered (VRI) CT images. The ostial narrowing of the left main coronary artery (LM) is seen in both images (arrows).

CHAPTER 4.1.2.2, REFERENCES 27, 90, 91

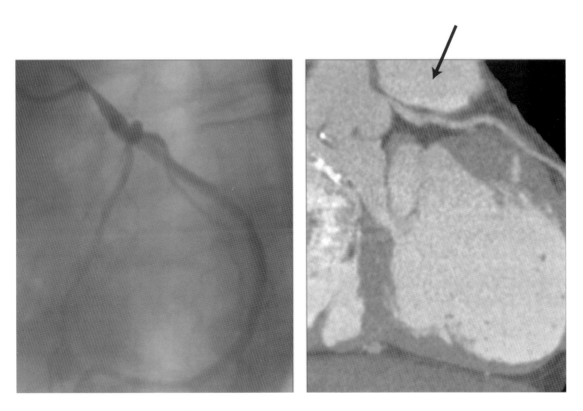

Figure 114 Left main compression (1.3)

Format: angiogram, MPR

The corresponding MPR image (right panel) again demonstrates the ostial narrowing. However, there is no associated atherosclerotic plaque accumulation of the left main. The pulmonary artery is prominent and appears to compress the left main coronary artery (arrow).

CHAPTER 4.1.2.2, REFERENCES 27, 90, 91

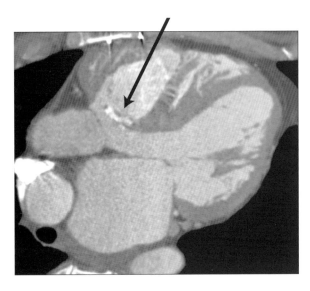 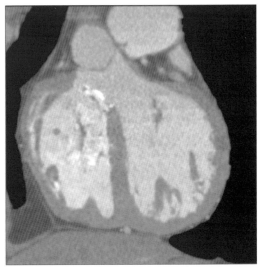

Figure 115   Left main compression (1.4)

Format: MPR

This figure demonstrates the cause of the dilated pulmonary artery. It shows evidence of remote repair of a VSD in the left ventricular outflow tract with surgical material (arrow). However, there is residual VSD with suspected shunting to the right ventricle and subsequent volume overload.

CHAPTER 4.1.2.2, REFERENCES 27, 90, 91

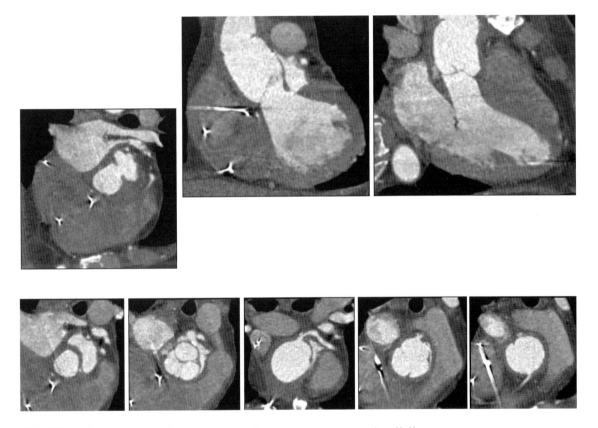

Figure 116 LV outflow tract pseudoaneurysm causing coronary compression (1.1)

Format: MPR

This figure shows images of a patient with a complicated history of repeat surgery for aortic valve disease, with eventual placement of a homograft. The patient presented with atypical chest pain, and a cardiac catheterization demonstrated systolic compression of the left main and left anterior descending coronary arteries (30–40% of luminal diameter).

The CT images show evidence of replacement of the ascending aorta with a homograft. There is wall thickening of the graft extending into the proximal segments of the reimplanted coronary arteries, compatible with inflammatory material. There is a pseudoaneurysm originating from the anterior left aspect of the left ventricular outflow tract below the aortic valve level. The cavity lies on the left side of the homograft and extends up to the level of the left main coronary artery ostium. The left main coronary artery and proximal LAD coronary artery are draped around the pseudoaneurysm cavity.

CHAPTER 4.1.2, REFERENCES 27, 90, 91

diastole   systole

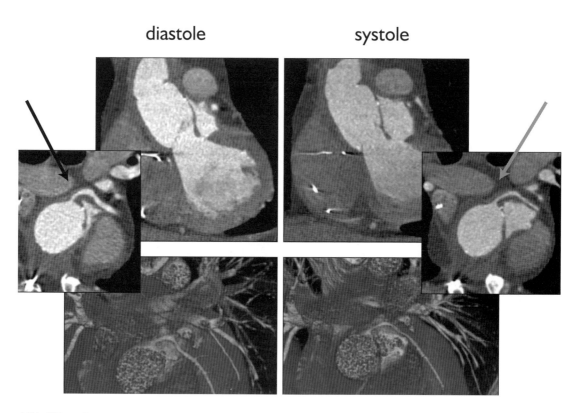

Figure 117   LV outflow tract pseudoaneurysm causing coronary compression (1.2) (see also color section on p. 10)

Format: MPR, VRI

The dimensions of the pseudoaneurysm are 2.5 × 3 × 3.5 cm in diastole and 3.6 × 4.0 × 3.8 cm in systole. This appears to be the cause of the systolic coronary compression of the left main coronary artery and proximal LAD coronary artery, which are draped around the cavity.

CHAPTER 4.1.2, REFERENCES 27, 90, 91

diastole   systole

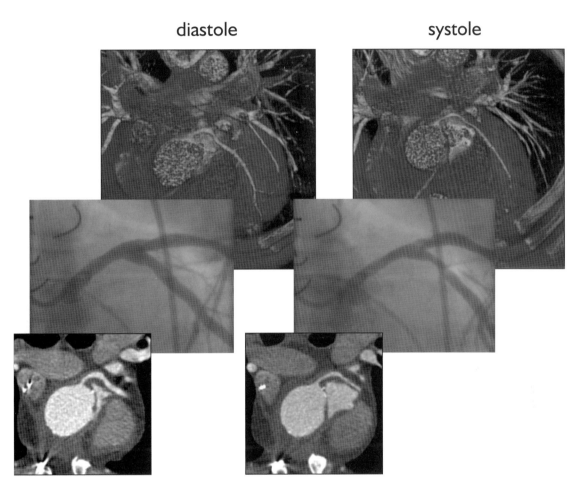

Figure 118   LV outflow tract pseudoaneurysm causing coronary compression (1.3) (see also color section on p. 11)

Format: MPR, VRI, angiogram

This figure shows a comparison of angiographic and CT images, demonstrating the systolic compression of the left main and left anterior descending coronary arteries.

CHAPTER 4.1.2, REFERENCES 27, 90, 91

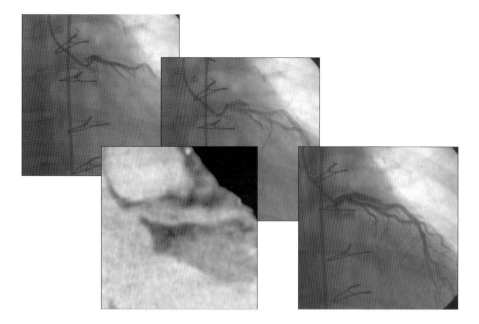

Figure 119 Left main dissection

Format: angiography, MPR

This figure shows angiographic and CT images of a patient with a chronic LM dissection and history of coronary bypass surgery with a LIMA graft to the LAD. The angiogram shows the dissection of the LM and proximal LAD. The CT image demonstrates enlargement of the left main coronary artery with irregular lumen size. The dissection flap can be seen.

CHAPTER 4.1.2.2, REFERENCES 27, 90, 91

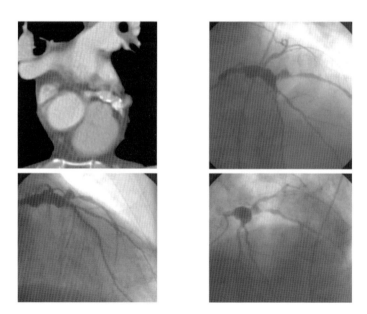

Figure 120 Coronary ectasia

Format: angiogram, MPR

Non-stenotic forms of atherosclerotic disease, including diffuse coronary ectasia and focal aneurysms can be assessed with CT.

This figure shows angiographic and CT images of a patient with a history of CAD and previous myocardial infarction. Both angiogram and CTA show ectasia of the proximal LAD consistent with mild aneurysm formation. There is calcification of the arterial wall.

CHAPTER 4.1.2.2, REFERENCES 27, 90, 91, 154

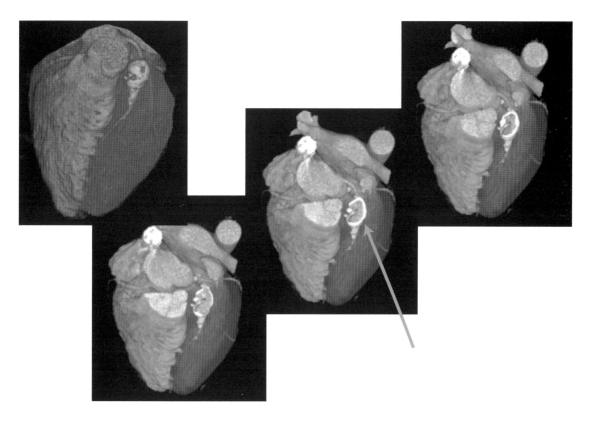

Figure 121   Left anterior descending coronary aneurysm (1.1) (see also color section on p. 11)

Format: VRI

This figure shows a focal aneurysm of the proximal LAD with extensive calcification of the aneurysm wall (arrow).

CHAPTER 4.1.2.2, REFERENCES 27, 90, 91, 154

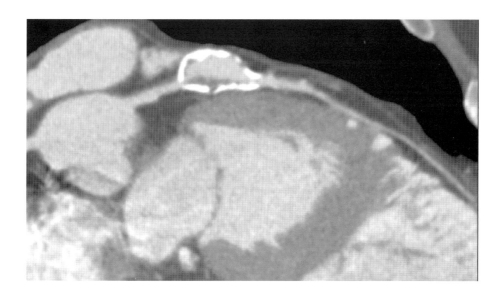

Figure 122   Left anterior descending coronary aneurysm (1.2)

Format: MPR

The MPR image shows the calcified wall of the aneurysm and a small amount of adherent wall thrombus inside the aneurysm.

CHAPTER 4.1.2.2, REFERENCES 27, 90, 91, 154

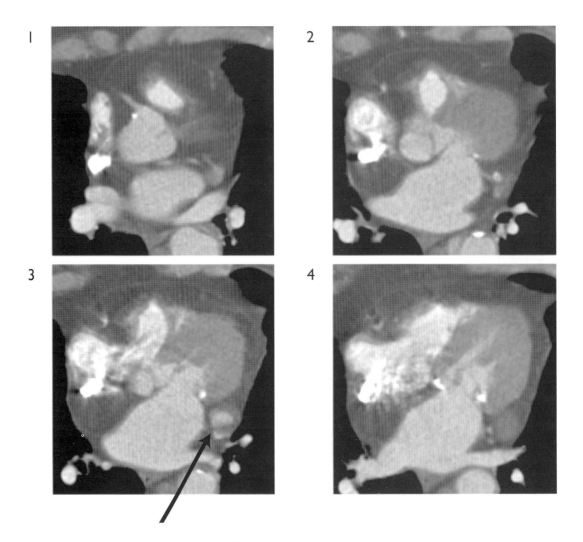

Figure 123 Left circumflex coronary aneurysm (1.1)

Format: MPR

An example of a focal aneurysm of the left circumflex coronary artery (LCX) is shown in these four axial images (cranial to caudal, 1–4). There is calcification of the LCX proximal to the aneurysm and a moderate amount of adherent wall thrombus inside the aneurysm (arrow).

CHAPTER 4.1.2.2, REFERENCES 27, 90, 91, 154

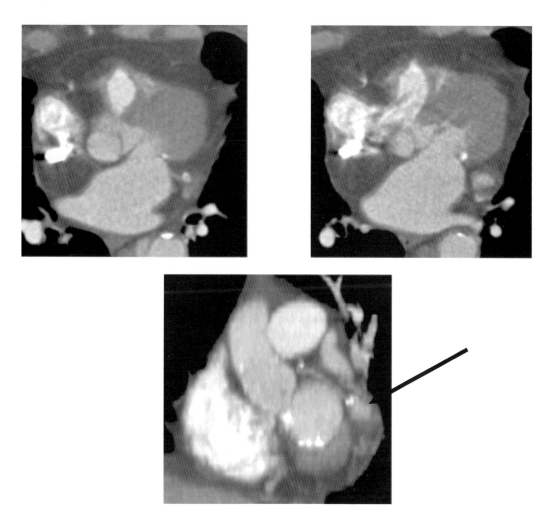

Figure 124 Left circumflex coronary aneurysm (1.2)

Format:: MPR

The location of the aneurysm is demonstrated on the oblique image (arrow, lower panel).

CHAPTER 4.1.2.2, REFERENCES 27, 90, 91, 154

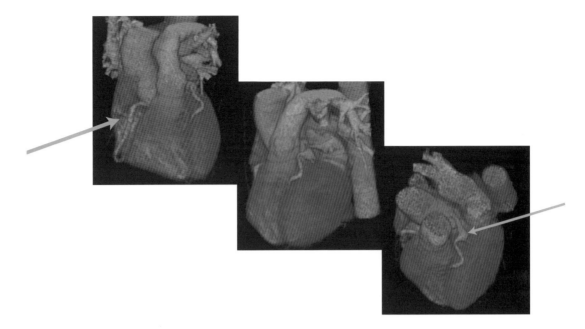

Figure 125 Diffuse coronary ectasia (1.1) (see also color section on p. 12)

Format: VRI

The images in this figure show a diffuse pattern of coronary ectasia, most notably involving the distal left main (thin arrow). The left main artery gives rise to a mildly ectatic left anterior descending coronary artery and a diminutive circumflex coronary artery. There is ectasia of the right coronary artery (thick arrow). No definite evidence of atherosclerotic changes of the coronary arteries is noted.

CHAPTER 4.1.2.2, REFERENCES 27, 90, 91, 154

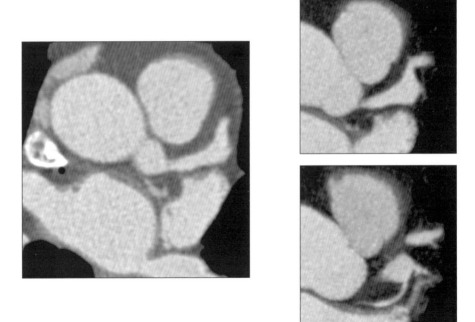

Figure 126 Coronary ectasia (1.2)

Format: MPR

The MPR images show the ectatic left main coronary artery (left panel) with the origins of the ectatic LAD (right upper panel) and diminutive LCX (right lower panel).

CHAPTER 4.1.2.2, REFERENCES 27, 90, 91, 154

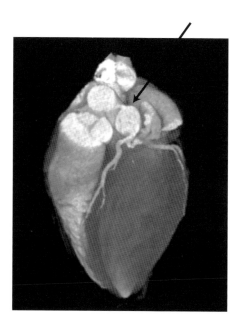

Figure 127   Left main coronary aneurysm

Format: VRI

Non-atherosclerotic aneurysmal disease is also seen with inflammatory diseases. This figure shows a large left main coronary artery aneurysm in a patient with a history of Kawasaki's disease (arrow).

CHAPTER 4.1.2.2, REFERENCES 27, 90, 91

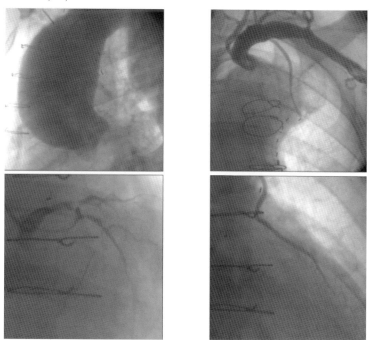

Figure 128   Bypass graft assessment (1.1)

Format: angiogram

The next figures (128–130) show angiographic and CT images of coronary bypass grafts. In this figure, the angiogram demonstrates severe disease of the proximal LAD and LCX (left lower panel). A patent LIMA graft to the LAD is demonstrated (right upper and right lower panels). There is aneurysmal dilatation of the ascending aorta (left upper panel). The aorto-coronary grafts originating at the dilated ascending aorta are not well seen because of poor contrast enhancement, and the patient was therefore referred for CT.

CHAPTER 4.1.2.2, REFERENCES 27, 90, 91, 155–160

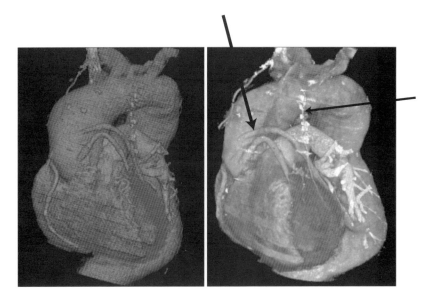

Figure 129 Bypass graft assessment (1.2) (see also color section on p. 12)

Format: VRI

This figure shows volume-rendered CT images of the dilated ascending aorta. The aorto-coronary bypass grafts to the LAD, LCX and RCA are demonstrated (thick arrow). A LIMA graft to the LAD is also shown (thin arrow). There is arrhythmia artifact (Figures 29 and 30) in the basal segments of the heart.

CHAPTER 4.1.2.2, REFERENCES 27, 90, 91, 155–160

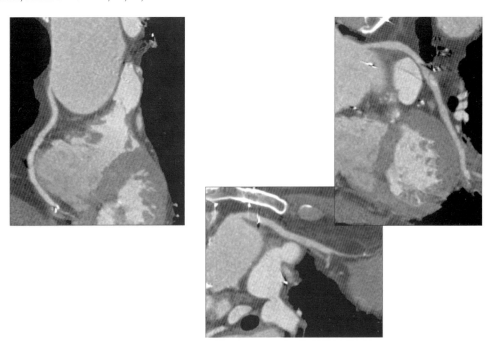

Figure 130 Bypass graft assessment (1.3)

Format: MPR

These MPR images demonstrate the bypass grafts. The aorto-coronary graft to the distal RCA has an area of focal narrowing approaching 50% at its origin (left upper panel). The graft extending to a major obtuse marginal branch of the circumflex coronary artery demonstrates no significant narrowing (right upper panel). The venous graft extending to the mid-LAD has diffuse areas of smooth insignificant narrowing.

CHAPTER 4.1.2.2, REFERENCES 27, 90, 91, 155–160

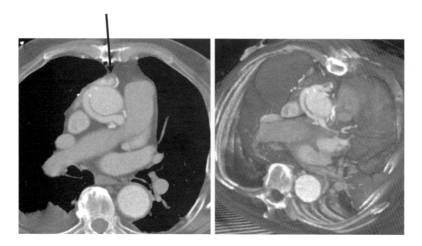

Figure 131 Reimplantation of coronary arteries with interposed graft

Format: MPR, VRI

This figure shows images of a patient with a remote history of aortic valve replacement, with valved conduit and reimplantation of the coronary arteries into the mid-portion of the valved conduit of the ascending aorta. There is an interposed graft originating above the right coronary cusp and immediately bifurcating into two limbs. One limb connects to the right coronary artery. There is a small aneurysmal dilatation at the anastomosis with the right coronary artery (arrow). The other limb takes a course behind the aorta and connects to the left main coronary artery. The graft and the proximal native coronary arteries are patent.

CHAPTER 4.1.2.2, REFERENCES 27, 90, 91, 155–160

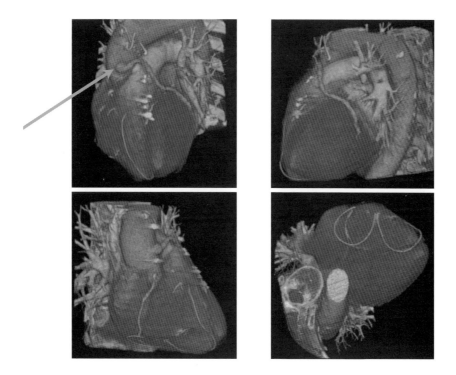

Figure 132 Stented bypass graft (1.1) (see also color section on p. 13)

Format: VRI

Because of their large size, stents in coronary bypass grafts can often be assessed for patency and severity of stenosis.
This figure shows images of a patient with a history of coronary artery bypass graft (CABG) and subsequent stenting of a focal stenosis in the proximal segment of the saphenous vein graft (SVG) to LCX. The stent location is demonstrated in these VRI images (arrow).

CHAPTER 4.1.2.2, REFERENCES 27, 90, 91, 155–160

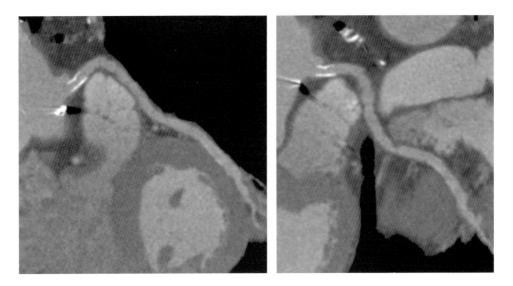

Figure 133   Stented bypass graft (1.2)

Format: MPR

These MPR images show the patent stent in the ostium of the aorto-coronary grafts.

CHAPTER 4.1.2.2, REFERENCES 27, 90, 91, 155–160

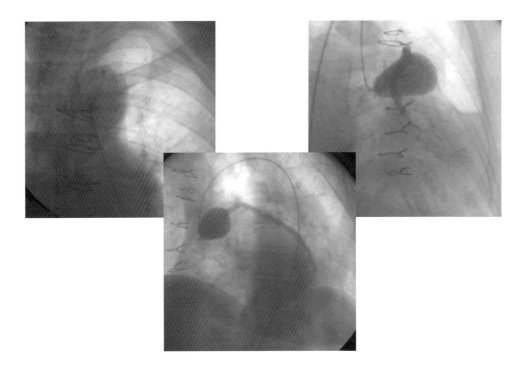

Figure 134   Bypass graft aneurysm (1.1)

Format: angiogram

The next images in Figures 134–139 demonstrate findings in a patient with a coronary bypass graft aneurysm. The angiogram shows a contrast-filled structure adjacent to the ascending thoracic aorta consistent with an aneurysm of an aorto-coronary graft to the circumflex coronary artery.

CHAPTER 4.1.2.2, REFERENCES 27, 90, 91, 155–160

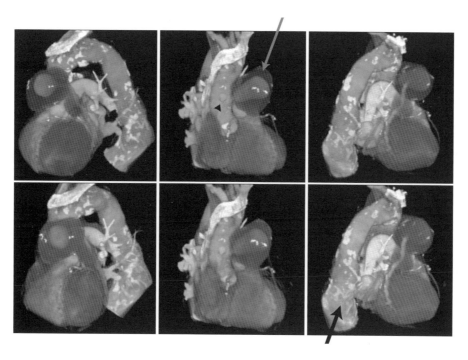

Figure 135   Bypass graft aneurysm (1.2)

Format: VRI

In this figure, corresponding volume-rendered CT images are shown. There is a patent saphenous vein graft to the circumflex artery, which is aneurysmally dilated in its proximal segments (thin arrow). The aneurysmally dilated segment at the origin of the graft is partially filled with thrombus, which surrounds the dilated contrast-filled lumen. Additional stumps of aorto-coronary grafts are seen in the ascending aorta (arrowhead). There is fusiform dilatation of the lower descending thoracic aorta with a maximum diameter of 5 cm (thick arrow).

CHAPTER 4.1.2.2, REFERENCES 27, 90, 91, 155–160

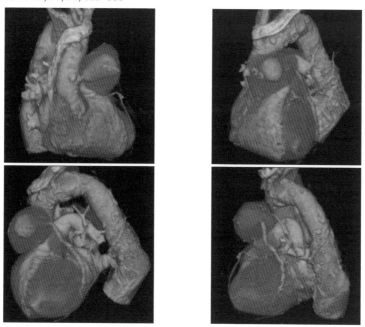

Figure 136   Bypass graft aneurysm (1.3) (see also color section on p. 13)

Format: VRI

The thrombus surrounding the contrast-filled dilated lumen is seen.

CHAPTER 4.1.2.2, REFERENCES 27, 90, 91, 155–160

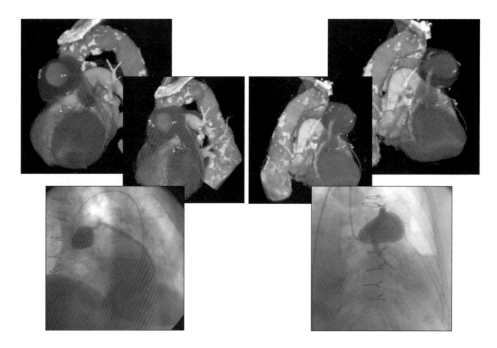

Figure 137   Bypass graft aneurysm (1.4)

Format: VRI, angiogram

Comparison between angiographic and CT images demonstrates the aneurysmally dilated segments in the proximal segments of the graft. The angiogram shows the perfused lumen, while the CT also shows the thrombus-filled aneurysm sac surrounding the contrast-filled lumen.

CHAPTER 4.1.2.2, REFERENCES 27, 90, 91, 155–160

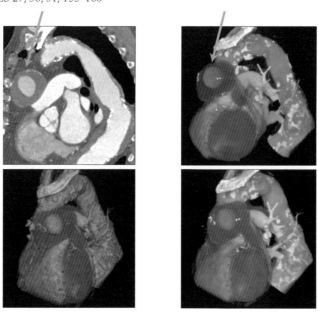

Figure 138   Bypass graft aneurysm (1.5) (see also color section on p. 14)

Format: MPR, VRI

Comparison between VRI and MPR images demonstrates the aneurysmally dilated segments (arrows). The aneurysmally dilated segment at the origin of the graft is partially filled with thrombus and measures 6.9 cm in its largest diameter. The luminal diameter reaches 4.3 cm in this segment.

CHAPTER 4.1.2.2, REFERENCES 27, 90, 91, 155–160

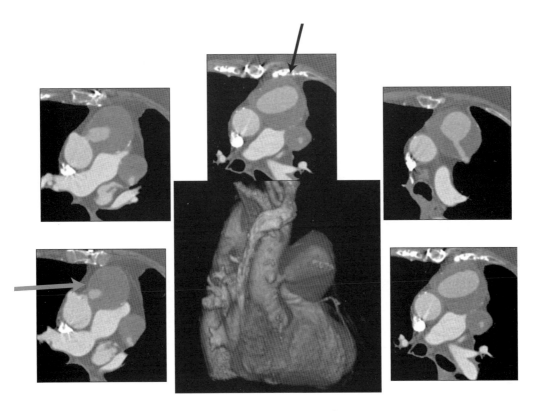

Figure 139 Bypass graft aneurysm (1.6) (see also color section on p. 14)

Format: MPR, VRI

These MPR images demonstrate the aneurysmally dilated segments. The aneurysmally dilated, partially thrombosed segment at the origin of the graft measures 6.9 cm in its largest diameter (arrows). The diameter of the contrast-filled lumen reaches 4.3 cm. There is a smaller aneurysmal dilatation measuring 3 cm, with normal luminal diameter. There is no evidence of luminal stenosis.

CHAPTER 4.1.2.2, REFERENCES 27, 90, 91, 155–160

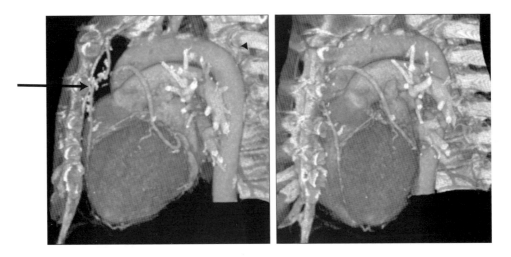

Figure 140 Location of bypass grafts (1.1)

Format: VRI

An important application is the assessment of graft position before repeat bypass surgery. As shown in this figure, knowledge about the proximity of the LIMA graft (arrow) to the sternum can help the surgeon in planning the approach. In addition to the LIMA graft to the LAD, there is an aorto-coronary jump graft to a diagonal branch of the LAD and the LCX.

CHAPTER 4.1.2.2, REFERENCES 27, 90, 91, 155–160

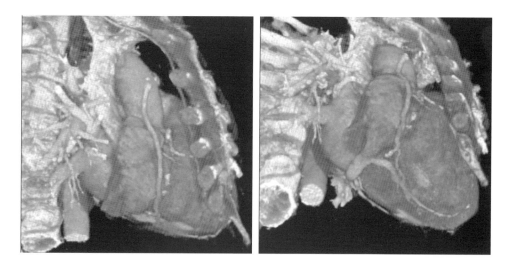

Figure 141   Location of bypass grafts (1.2)

Format: VRI

In addition, there is an aorto-coronary graft to the RCA.

CHAPTER 4.1.2.2, REFERENCES 27, 90, 91, 155–160

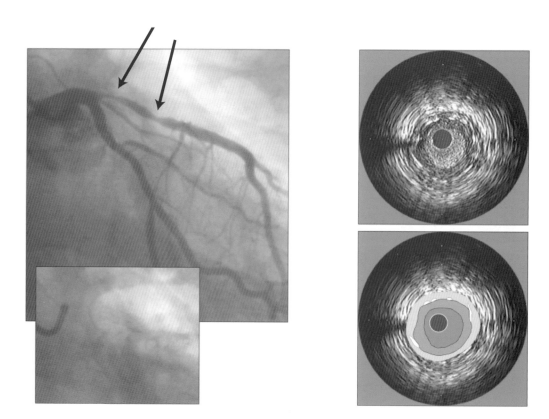

Figure 142   Coronary stent (1.1) (see also color section on p. 15)

Format: angiogram, intravascular ultrasound (IVUS)

The high-density metallic mesh of coronary stents precludes confident detection and grading of in-stent restenosis with CT. This figure shows angiographic and intravascular ultrasound images of a patient with moderate in-stent restenosis and severe stenosis at the stent edges (arrows).

CHAPTER 4.1.2.2, REFERENCES 161–163

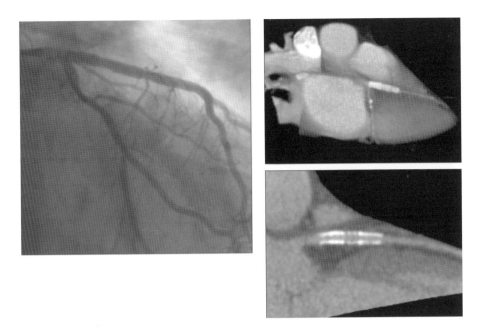

Figure 143   Coronary stent (1.2)

Format: angiogram, MPR, VRI

The patient underwent repeat percutaneous coronary intervention with placement of overlapping proximal and distal stents. A post-interventional angiogram and corresponding CT images are shown. The overlapping stents are seen (right lower panel). However, precise assessment of luminal dimensions inside the stents is limited with CT, secondary to the blooming artifact of the stent struts.

CHAPTER 4.1.2.2, REFERENCES 161–163

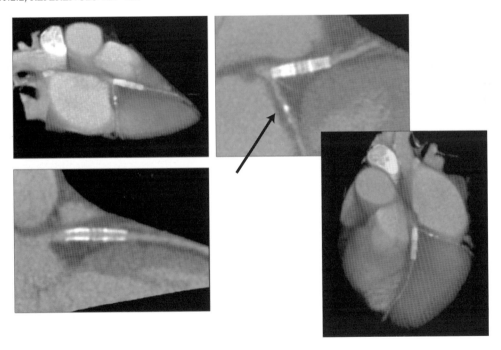

Figure 144   Coronary stent (1.3)

Format: MPR, VRI

CT demonstrates the exact location of the stent in relation to the left main bifurcation. In addition, calcified plaque is demonstrated in the LCX (arrow).

CHAPTER 4.1.2.2, REFERENCES 161–163

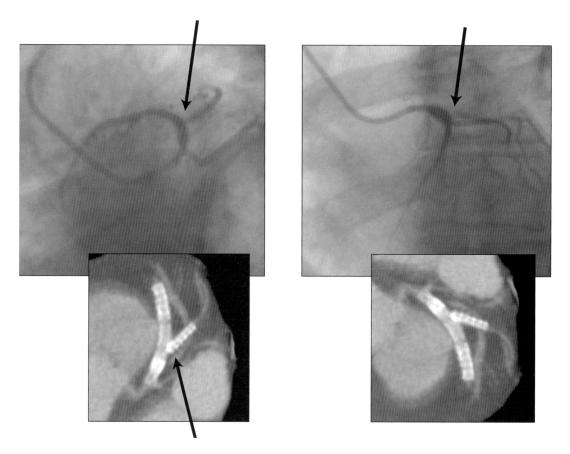

Figure 145 Coronary stent

Format: MPR, angiogram

This figure shows pre-interventional angiographic and CT images of a patient with in-stent restensosis of a previous stent deployed in the first diagonal branch of the LAD (arrows). There are additional patent stents in the proximal LAD. Because of the small size of the stent, the stenotic lumen cannot be reliably assessed with CT.

CHAPTER 4.1.2.2, REFERENCES 161–163

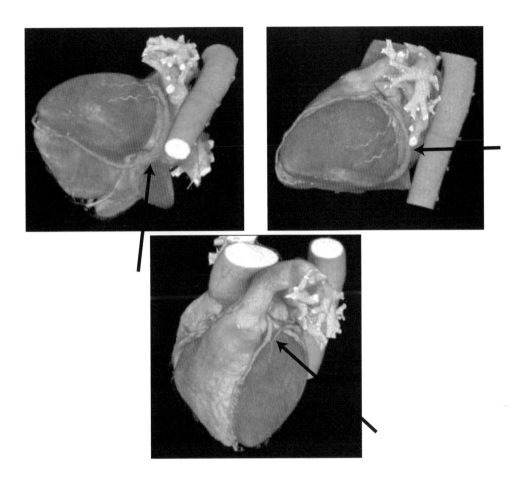

Figure 146 Coronary sinus

Format: VRI

Because of the intravenous rather than selective arterial contrast injection, the coronary sinus and coronary veins are typically faintly enlarged in CT images but not in angiograms. Because of their course partially parallel to arteries, veins can be mistaken for coronary arteries. If venous structures are the primary focus of the examination, then slightly different contrast timing or multiphasic imaging (arterial and venous phases) is often performed.

In this figure, normal vein anatomy is shown. The great cardiac vein runs parallel to the proximal LAD (lower panel, arrow), then follows the LCX into the atrioventricular groove (right upper panel, arrow) and drains into the right atrium as the coronary sinus (left upper panel, arrow).

CHAPTER 4.1.3, REFERENCES 164, 165

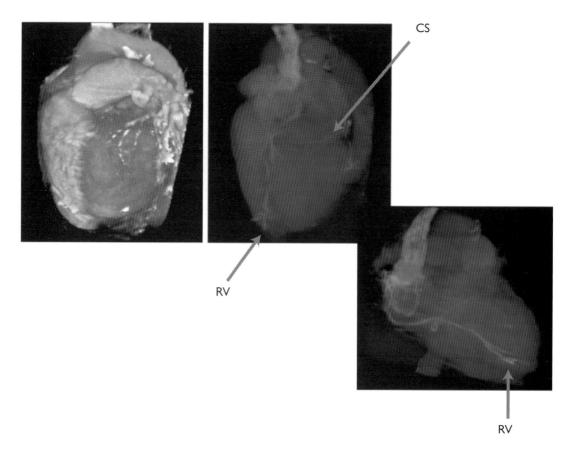

Figure 147   Biventricular pacemaker lead in coronary sinus

Format: VRI

A recent clinical question is assessment of coronary sinus anatomy for placement or checking of pacer lead position. In this figure, pacer leads of a biventricular pacing lead are visible in the right ventricle (RV) and coronary sinus (CS) (arrows).

CHAPTER 4.1.3, REFERENCES 164, 165

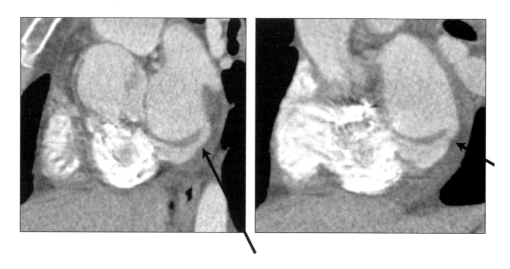

Figure 148   Coronary sinus fistula

Format: MPR

This figure shows a fistula connecting the coronary sinus and left atrium (arrows).

CHAPTER 4.1.3, REFERENCES 165

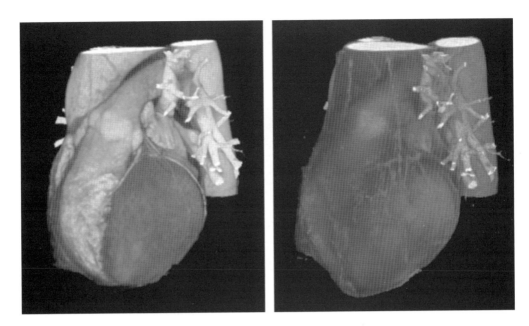

Figure 149 Normal pericardium (1.1)

Format: VRI

The normal pericardium, which has a thickness of 1–2 mm, can be delineated over the left and right ventricles. By changing opacity in this volume-rendered image, the heart is seen with (right panel) and without (left panel) the normal pericardium. The thin pericardial sac wraps the ventricles, the coronary arteries and the root of the aorta.

CHAPTER 4.1.4, REFERENCES 166–168

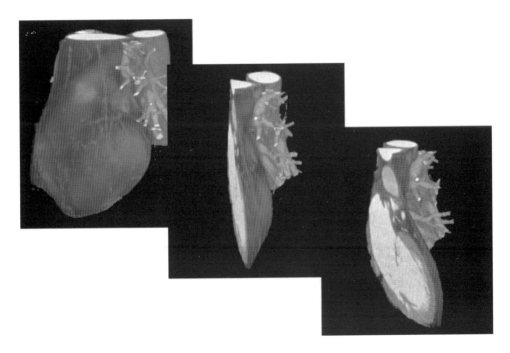

Figure 150 Normal pericardium (1.2)

Format: VRI

Further manipulation of the volume-rendered image demonstrates the location of the pericardial sac wrapping the ventricles and the coronary arteries.

CHAPTER 4.1.4, REFERENCES 166–168

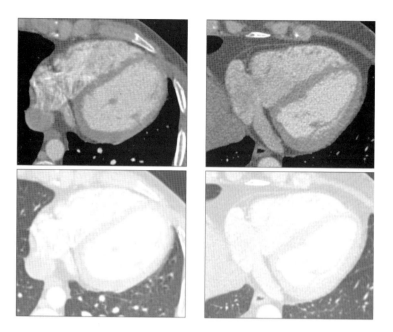

Figure 151   Normal and absent pericardium (1.1)

Format: MPR

MDCT delineates the pericardium over the left and right ventricles. Congenital or post-surgical absence of the pericardium can be identified.

This figure compares normal pericardial anatomy (right panels) with congenital absence of the pericardium (left panels). The relationship of the lungs, the pericardial fat and the pericardium is shown. The image settings in the upper panels are optimized for soft tissue, the lower panels for lung tissue ('lung windows').

CHAPTER 4.1.4, REFERENCES 166–168

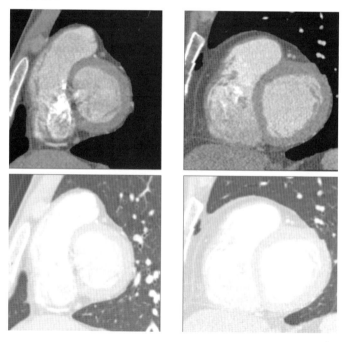

Figure 152   Normal and absent pericardium (1.2)

Format: MPR

The corresponding short-axis views of the left and right ventricles clearly show the missing structure of the pericardium. The image settings in the upper panels are optimized for soft tissue, the lower panels for lung tissue ('lung windows').

CHAPTER 4.1.4, REFERENCES 166–168

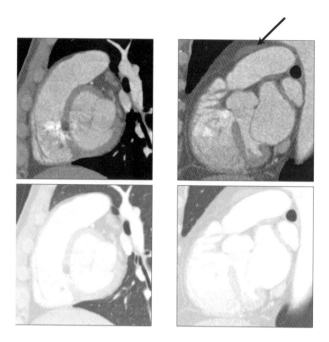

Figure 153 Normal and absent pericardium (1.3)

Format: MPR

In the same patient, this figure demonstrates the extension of the pericardium to the proximal right ventricular outflow tract (arrow). The image settings in the upper panels are optimized for soft tissue, the lower panels for lung tissue ('lung windows').

CHAPTER 4.1.4, REFERENCES 166–168

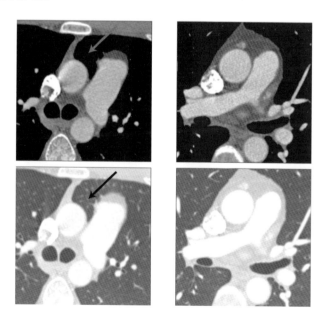

Figure 154 Normal and absent pericardium (1.4)

Format: MPR

Because the normal pericardium extends to the proximal ascending aorta, the recess between the aorta and the pulmonary artery provides further clues to the absence of the pericardium. As shown in this figure, this recess is filled by lung tissue in the patient with absence of the pericardium (arrows). The image settings in the upper panels are optimized for soft tissue, the lower panels for lung tissue ('lung windows').

CHAPTER 4.1.4, REFERENCES 166–168

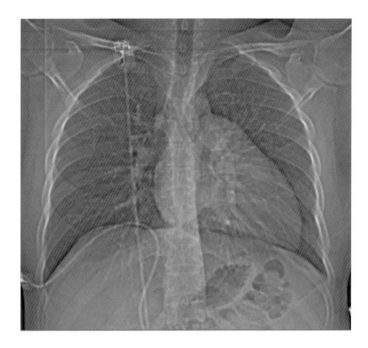

Figure 155   Absent pericardium (2.1)

Format: planar chest X-ray

Another example of congenital absence of the pericardium is shown in this and the following images. The chest X-ray shows the typical features of an absent pericardium.

CHAPTER 4.1.4, REFERENCES 166–168

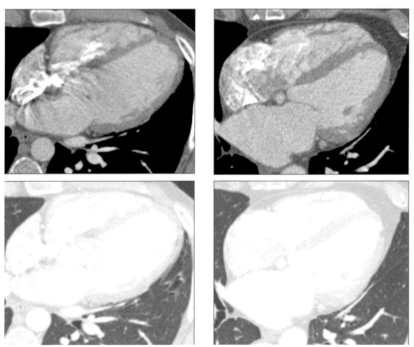

Figure 156   Absent pericardium (2.2)

Format: MPR

The corresponding CT of a four-chamber view (left panels) is shown in comparison with a patient with normal pericardium (right panels). The image settings in the upper panels are optimized for soft tissue, the lower panels for lung tissue ('lung windows').

CHAPTER 4.1.4, REFERENCES 166–168

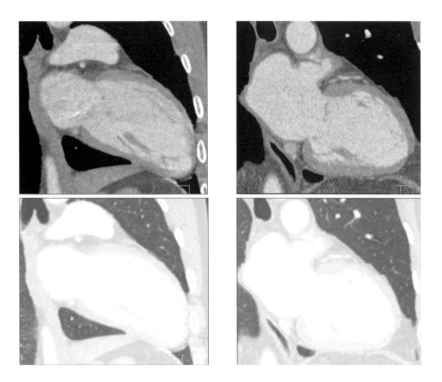

Figure 157   Absent pericardium (2.3)

Format: MPR

This figure shows the corresponding two-chamber views. The image settings in the upper panels are optimized for soft tissue, the lower panels for lung tissue ('lung windows').

CHAPTER 4.1.4, REFERENCES 166–168

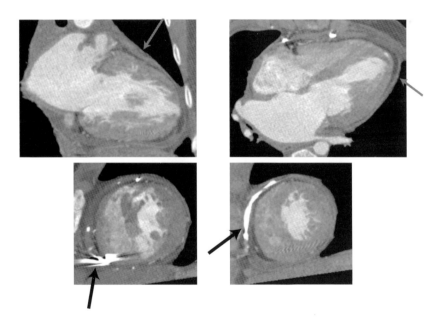

Figure 158   Pericardial thickening

Format: MPR

MDCT can reliably demonstrate pericardial thickening. This figure demonstrates circumferential thickening of the pericardium (thin arrows). An epicardial pacer wire is seen adjacent to the right ventricle (thick arrows).

CHAPTER 4.1.4, REFERENCES 166–168

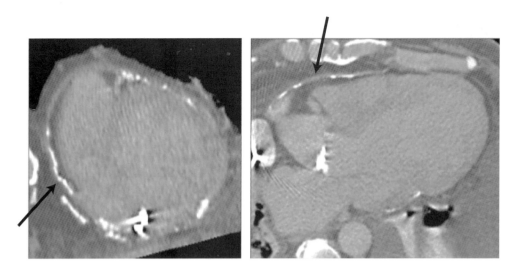

Figure 159 Thickened pericardium with calcification (1)

Format: MPR

In this non-contrast-enhanced CT scan, circumferential mild thickening of the pericardium is associated with mild calcification (arrows).

CHAPTER 4.1.4, REFERENCES 166–168

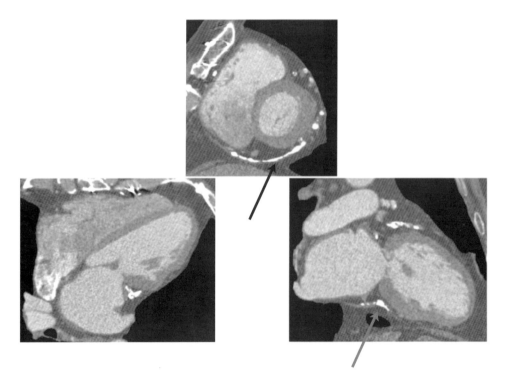

Figure 160 Pericardial calcification (2.1)

Format: MPR

The images in this figure show extensive focal pericardial calcification over the basal inferior wall of the heart (arrows). The patient has a remote history of coronary bypass surgery.

CHAPTER 4.1.4, REFERENCES 166–168

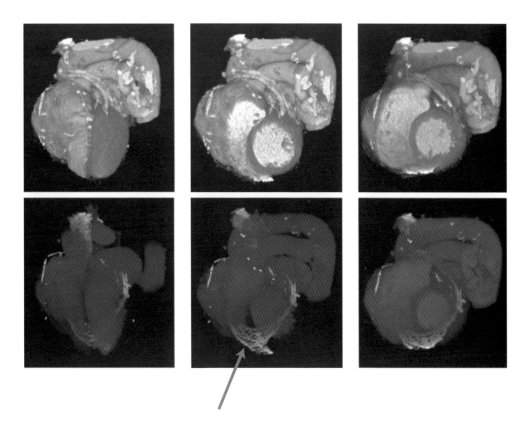

Figure 161   Pericardial calcification (2.2)

Format: VRI

This figure shows volume-reduced images with regular image settings (upper panels) and with faded soft tissues (lower panels). The wedge-shaped calcification at the base of the heart is seen (arrow). Several bypass grafts are demonstrated in the left upper panel.

CHAPTER 4.1.4, REFERENCES 166–168

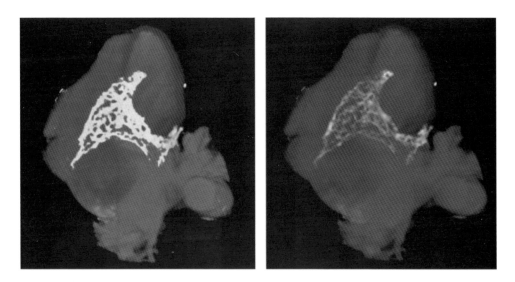

Figure 162   Pericardial calcification (2.3)

Format: VRI

The location of the calcification is shown in these volume-rendered images showing the base of the heart.

CHAPTER 4.1.4, REFERENCES 166–168

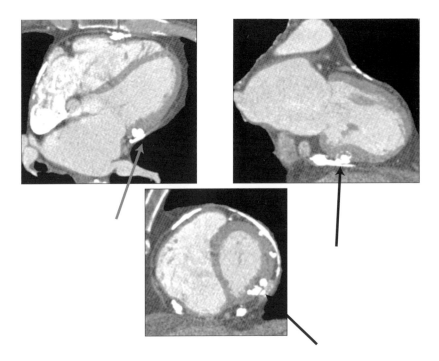

Figure 163   Pericardial calcification (3.1)

Format: MPR

Images of another patient with extensive calcification of the pericardium are shown in this figure. Calcification of the posterolateral wall appears to extend into the myocardium (arrows).

CHAPTER 4.1.4, REFERENCES 166–168

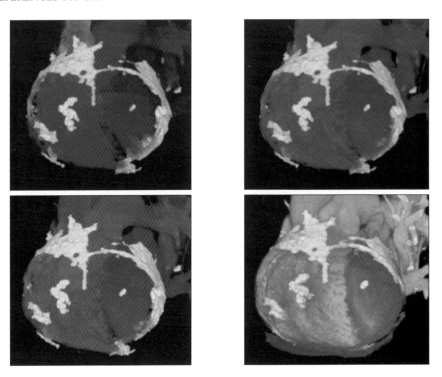

Figure 164   Pericardial calcification (3.2)

Format: VRI

The volume-rendered images clearly show the extent and location of the calcification.

CHAPTER 4.1.4, REFERENCES 166–168

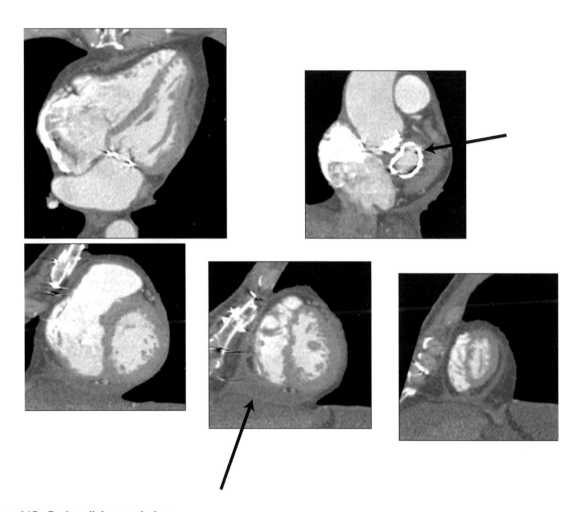

Figure 165   Pericardial constriction

Format: MPR

The detection of increased pericardial thickness, especially with pericardial calcium, in combination with conical/tubular deformation of the ventricles, provides evidence of pericardial constriction.

This figure shows images of a patient with a remote history of mitral valve repair using a prosthetic ring (arrow, right upper panel). There is diffuse circumferential thickening of the pericardium measuring up to 5 mm. There is a small amount of pericardial effusion, localized predominantly over the inferior aspect of the right ventricle (arrow, lower middle panel). There is tubular deformation of the normal-size left and right ventricles (upper left panel). These findings are consistent with pericardial constriction.

CHAPTER 4.1.4, REFERENCES 166–168

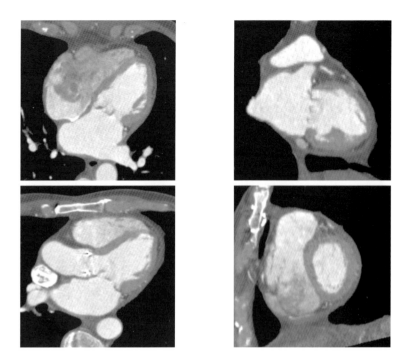

Figure 166 Pericardial constriction

Format: MPR

However, while thickening and calcification of the pericardium is a reliable sign of pericardial disease, it does not prove the presence of constrictive physiology, which is best assessed with echocardiography or MRI.

This figure shows images of a patient with a history of aortic valve replacement. The pericardium appears thickened although not calcified. The maximal thickness is 4 mm. There is mild conical deformation of the left ventricle. Echocardiography was consistent with constrictive physiology.

CHAPTER 4.1.4, REFERENCES 166–168

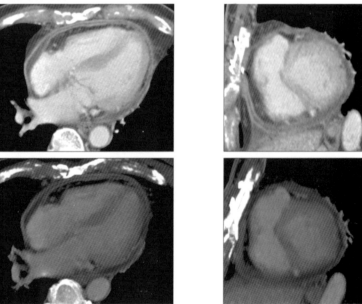

Figure 167 Pericardial enhancement (1)

Format: MPR, MIP

CT scans after contrast administration can provide information about the possible inflammatory nature of a pericardial process. Contrast enhancement of the pericardial layers, as shown in this figure, is consistent with pericarditis.

CHAPTER 4.1.4, REFERENCES 166–168

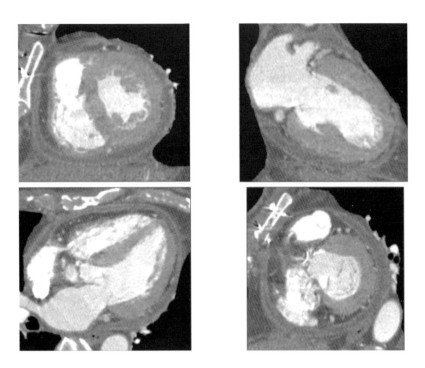

Figure 168   Pericarditis (2)

Format: MPR

Another example of thickening and contrast enhancement of both the parietal and the visceral pericardium with a small pericardial effusion is shown in this figure. The findings are consistent with pericarditis.

CHAPTER 4.1.4, REFERENCES 166–168

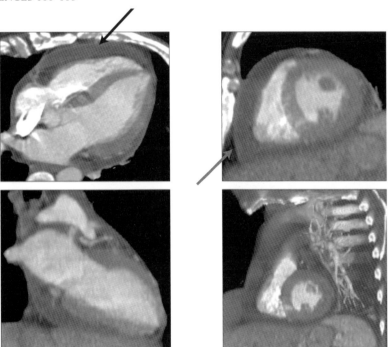

Figure 169   Pericarditis (3)

Format: MPR, VRI

In these images, pericardial enhancement is associated with a small-to-moderate size circumferential pericardial effusion (arrows).

CHAPTER 4.1.4, REFERENCES 166–168

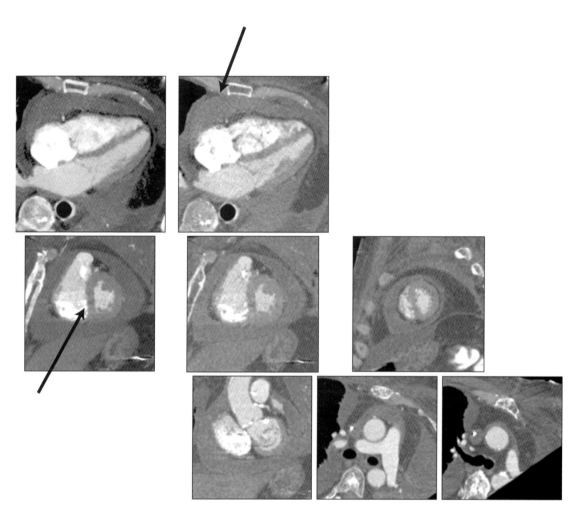

Figure 170 Pericardial effusion (1)

Format: MPR, MIP

CT allows identification of the amount and characteristics of pericardial fluid adjacent to the right and left ventricles. The images in this figure show normal pericardial thickness with a moderate-to-large pericardial effusion (arrow, right upper panel). The patient presented with shortness of breath 1 month after initiation of coumadin therapy. There is straightening of the interventricular septum (arrow, left middle panel) and tubular deformity of the left ventricle (left upper panel), suggesting a component of pericardial constriction. The right ventricle is mildly dilated, without evidence of tamponade. Subsequently, surgical pericardectomy was performed. During surgery, a partially organized 1-inch (2.5 cm) thick layer of circumferential thrombus was removed.

CHAPTER 4.1.4, REFERENCES 166–168

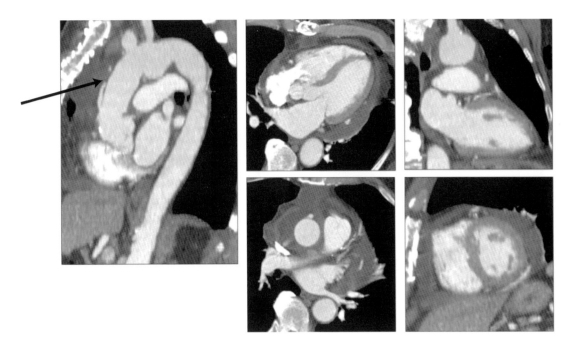

Figure 171 Postoperative pericardial effusion (2)

Format: MIP

This figure shows images of a patient after replacement of the ascending aorta. A supracoronary graft of the ascending aorta is seen (arrow, left panel). There is a small-to-moderate sized circumferential pericardial effusion without evidence of tamponade.

CHAPTER 4.1.4, REFERENCES 166–168

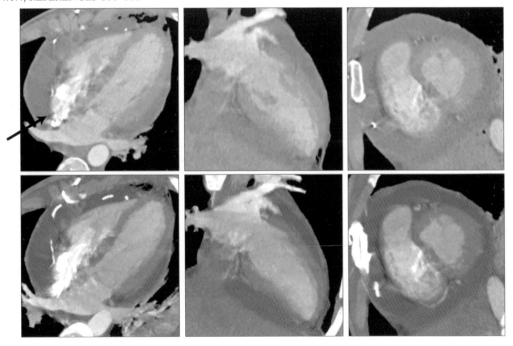

Figure 172 Pericardial tamponade

Format: MPR, MIP

This figure shows images of a patient with recent open heart surgery for replacement of the aortic root. There is a large pericardial effusion, with compression of the right atrium (arrow). In addition, dilatation of the inferior vena cava was seen. These findings are consistent with tamponade.

CHAPTER 4.1.4, REFERENCES 166–168

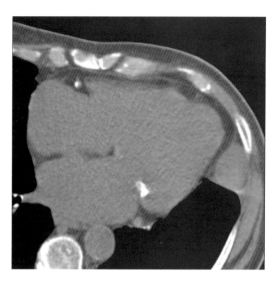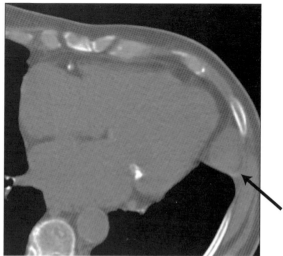

Figure 173   Pericardial cyst (1)

Format: MPR, MIP

In this non-contrast-enhanced CT scan an apical pericardial cyst is identified (arrow).

CHAPTER 4.1.4, REFERENCES 166–168

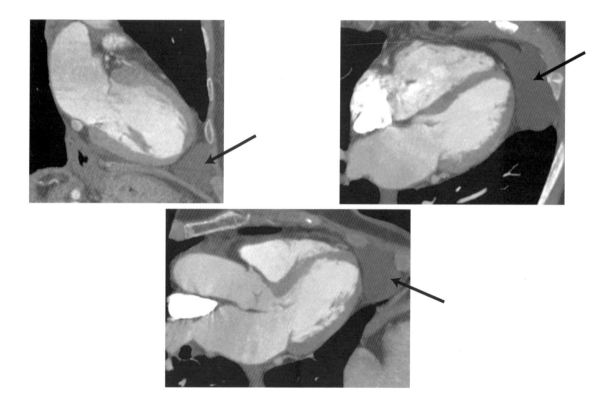

Figure 174   Pericardial cyst (2)

Format: MPR, MIP

A larger pericardial cyst over the left ventricular apex is shown (arrows). Contrast-enhanced scans help in the differentiation between cyst and normal ventricular cavity.

CHAPTER 4.1.4, REFERENCES 166–168

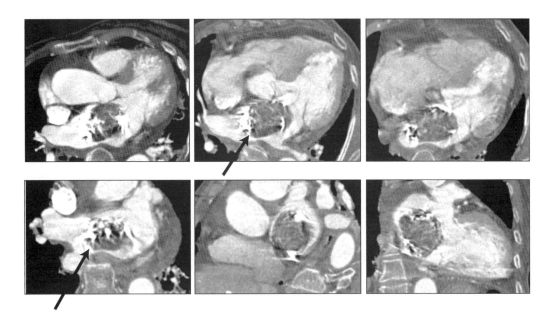

Figure 175 Suspected atrial myxoma (1)

Format: MPR, MIP

Atrial myxomas are common benign tumors. Myxomas often originate from the left atrium or mitral annulus with a stalk, and demonstrate tumor calcification.

This figure shows a large tumor in the left atrium, attached with a broad base to the intra-atrial septum (arrows). The tumor is partially calcified. The findings are suggestive of atrial myxoma.

CHAPTER 4.1.5,REFERENCES 169, 170

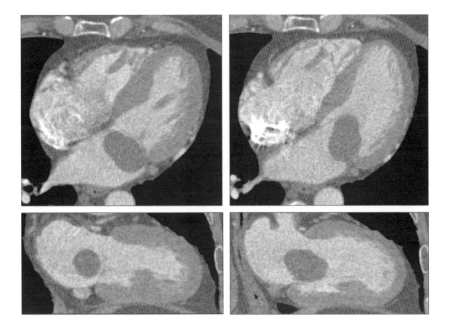

Figure 176 Atrial myxoma (2.1)

Format: MPR

Another example of a tumor with findings consistent with a myxoma is shown in this figure. There is a mass, which appears to be broadly attached to the posterior aspect of the mitral annulus and measures 2.8 × 2.8 × 3.7 cm. It is non-calcified and homogeneous and shows no evidence of enhancement.

CHAPTER 4.1.5, REFERENCES 169, 170

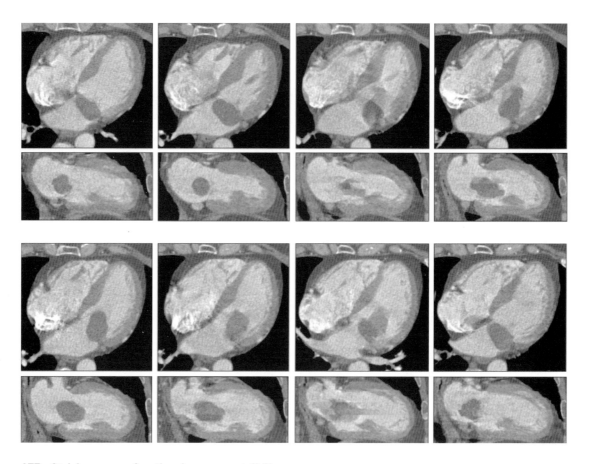

Figure 177   Atrial myxoma, functional assessment (2.2)

Format: MPR

This figure shows multiple reconstructions at different phases of the cardiac cycle. The images demonstrate that the mobile tumor passes through the valve plane during diastole (Movies 1 and 2).

CHAPTER 4.1.5, REFERENCES 169, 170

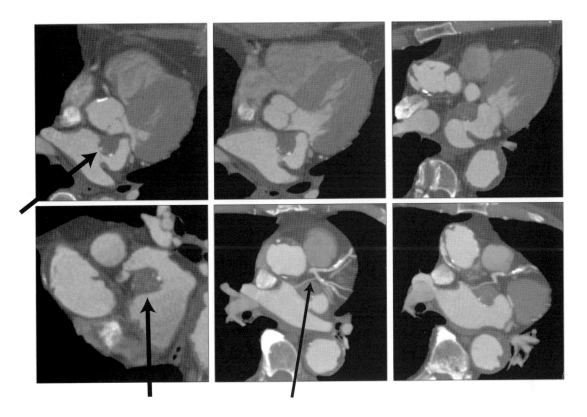

Figure 178 Suspected atrial myxoma

Format: MIP

However, definitive characterization of tumors is often not possible with CT imaging alone.

This figure shows a tumor contiguous with the roof of the left atrial body near the origin of the atrial appendage (thick arrows). The tissue is slightly heterogeneous with internal calcification and mild enhancement, measuring 2.0 × 1.6 × 1.7 cm. Originating form the proximal circumflex artery is an atrial branch which extends into the region of the mass of the left atrium (thin arrow). Although these findings are most consistent with atrial myxoma with atypical location, definitive characterization is not possible.

CHAPTER 4.1.5, REFERENCES 169, 170

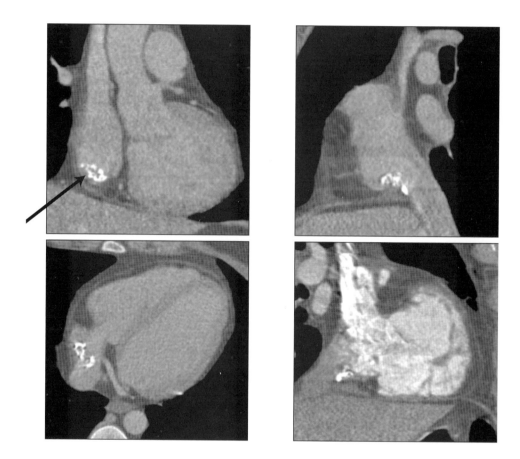

Figure 179   Calcified right atrial thrombus

Format: MPR

This figure shows images of a patient with a history of Hodgkin's disease. Image acquisition was delayed in relation to the contrast injection to avoid contrast artifacts in the right atrium (see Figure 15). At the inferior wall of the right atrium close to the junction with the inferior vena cava is a small tissue mound, which extends over a distance of 2 cm and has a thickness of 0.8 cm (arrow). There is calcification of the tissue.

The appearance suggests a benign process, most likely a calcified thrombus, secondary to trauma from a central line.

CHAPTER 4.1.5, REFERENCES 169, 170

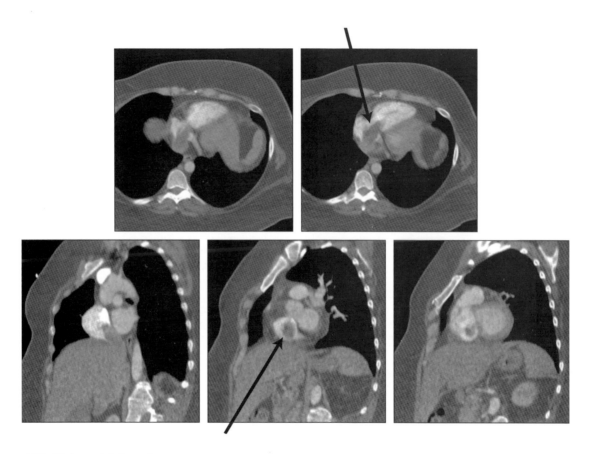

Figure 180   Right atrial thrombus

Format: MIP

This figure shows images of a low-density mass extending from the level of the upper inferior vena cava (IVC) near the confluence of the hepatic veins to the level of the tricuspid valve (arrows). The mass does not appear to occlude the IVC or the right-sided atrioventricular inflow. Its low attenuation suggests thrombus. The cardiac chambers are otherwise unremarkable. The kidneys are intact and there is no evidence of renal malignancy.

The patient underwent excision of the mass. Pathology was consistent with an organizing thrombus.

CHAPTER 4.1.5, REFERENCES 169, 170

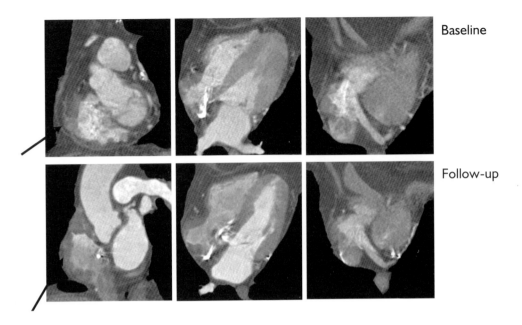

Baseline

Follow-up

Figure 181   Right atrial wall tumor

Format: MPR

This figure shows images of a patient at two different times, 6 months apart. There is lobular thickening involving the entire right atrium (arrows). The findings were thought to be consistent with benign hamartoma of the right atrium, and biopsy or surgery was deferred. At follow-up (lower panels) the mass was unchanged in thickness and appearance. Follow-up imaging demonstrating stability of the findings over time supports the likelihood of a benign nature.

CHAPTER 4.1.5, REFERENCES 169, 170

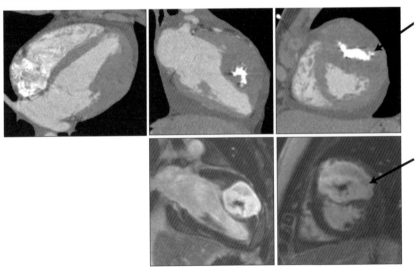

Figure 182   Suspected left ventricular fibroma

Format: MIP, MRI

An example of a suspected left ventricular fibroma is shown in this figure. CT images (upper panels) and MRI views (lower panels) are shown in comparison.

Within the anteroapical region of the left ventricle, beginning at the junction of the basal and middle one-third and occupying primarily the anterior wall but with extension into the anteroseptal and high-lateral regions, there is a mass measuring 4 × 4.7 × 5.8 cm (arrows). The lesion is well circumscribed without evidence of surrounding edema or neovascularity. The findings suggest dense fibrotic tissue with focal areas of calcification.

The patient subsequently underwent surgery with excision of the mass. Pathology confirmed the diagnosis of a cardiac fibroma.

CHAPTER 4.1.5, REFERENCES 169, 170

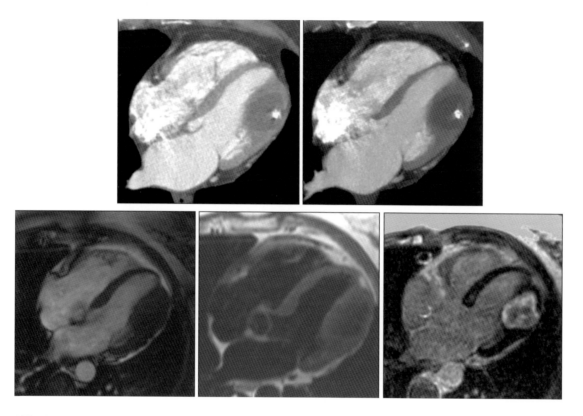

Figure 183 Suspected left ventricular fibroma

Format: MPR, MRI

Another tumor with similar characteristics is shown in this figure. CT images (upper panels) and MRI views (lower panels) are shown in comparison.
Based on the findings, a fibroma of the left ventricle was suspected.

CHAPTER 4.1.5, REFERENCES 169, 170

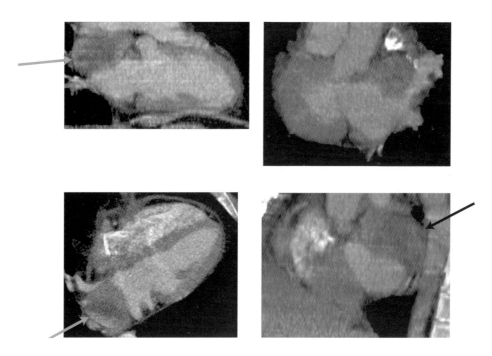

Figure 184   Left atrial paraganglioma (1.1)

Format: MIP

This and the next figure show pre- and postoperative images of a tumor at the roof of the left atrium (arrows). The patient underwent surgery and an intraoperative biopsy was consistent with an intrapericardial paraganglioma situated on the roof of the left atrium. The tumor was subsequently removed.

CHAPTER 4.1.5, REFERENCES: 169, 170

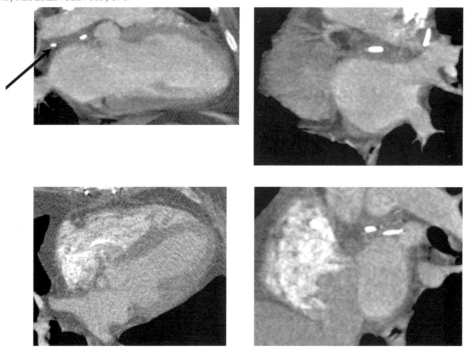

Figure 185   Left atrial paraganglioma (1.2)

Format: MPR

Images at follow-up did not show evidence of residual or recurrent tumor. Surgical clips are seen in the operative field (arrow).

CHAPTER 4.1.5, REFERENCES 169, 170

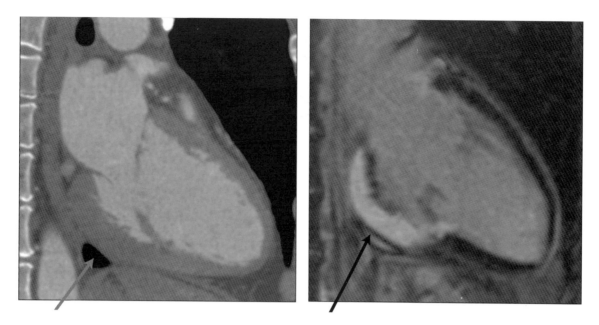

Figure 186   Suspected fibrosarcoma (1.1)

Format: MPR, MRI

A tumor of the inferior wall of the left ventricle is shown. There is infiltration of the myocardial wall, which is clearly shown with delayed contrast-enhanced MRI (arrow, right panel). The same area is less enhanced on the MDCT study. However, the hypoenhancement is not well seen on the MPR image (arrow, left panel).

CHAPTER 4.1.5, REFERENCES 169, 170

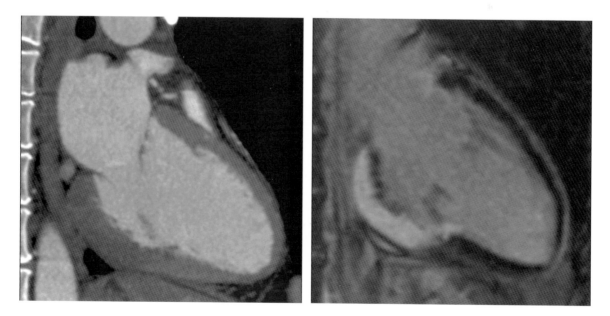

Figure 187   Suspected fibrosarcoma (1.2)

Format: MIP, MRI

The hypoenhancement of the inferior wall is better seen on the MIP image (left panel), but delayed contrast-enhanced MRI is clearly superior (right panel).

CHAPTER 4.1.5, REFERENCES 169, 170

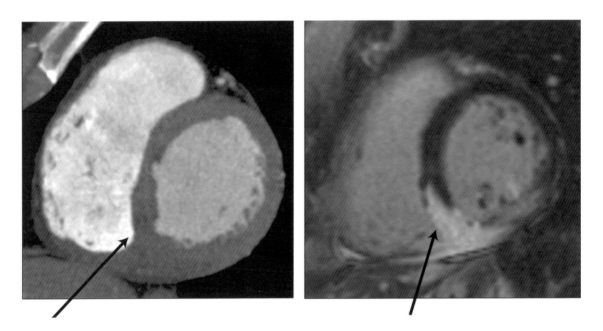

Figure 188   Suspected fibrosarcoma (1.3)

Format: MIP, MRI

The short-axis view demonstrates the location of the tumor of the left ventricle, extending into the right ventricle. Tissue infiltration is seen on the MIP image (arrow, left panel) and the delayed contrast-enhanced MRI view (arrow, right panel).

CHAPTER 4.1.5, REFERENCES 169, 170

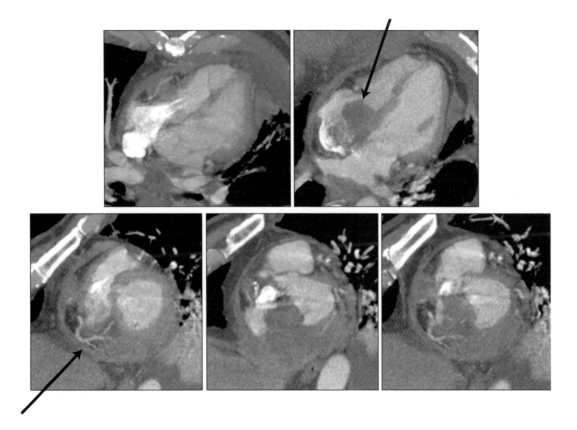

Figure 189   Right atrial spindle-cell sarcoma

Format: MIP

The figure shows a tumor of the right atrium (arrow, right upper panel). Several small tumor vessels are seen extending into the lesion (arrow, left lower panel). The patient underwent surgery with removal of the tumor. Pathology was consistent with a high-grade spindle-cell carcinoma.

CHAPTER 4.1.5, REFERENCES 169, 170

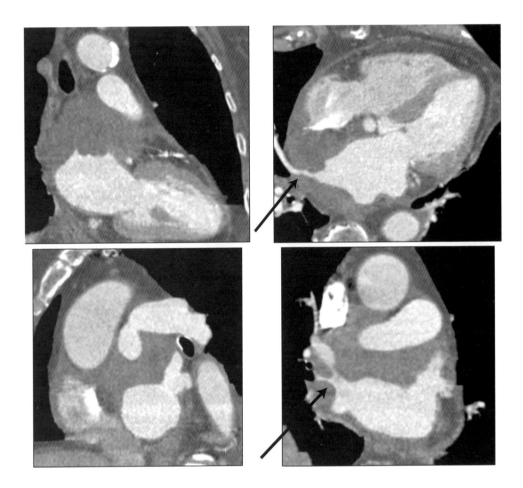

Figure 190   Cardiac lymphoma

Format: MIP

This figure shows images of a patient with lymphoma. There were mediastinal lymph nodes. There is a large mediastinal tumor with predominantly intrapericardial location. It involves the intra-atrial septum and the posterior and superior walls of the left and right atria. The tumor encases the pulmonary veins, with partial compression of the right superior vein ostium (arrows, right upper and lower panels). In addition, the tumor encases the superior vena cava, left main coronary artery, proximal left anterior descending artery and proximal left circumflex artery without causing significant compression.

During surgery a mass was found in the area of the aorta, right atrium and superior vena cava. The mass was densely adherent and infiltrative in the surrounding structures. Pathology was consistent with a diffuse, primary, mediastinal, large B-cell lymphoma.

CHAPTER 4.1.5, REFERENCES 169, 170

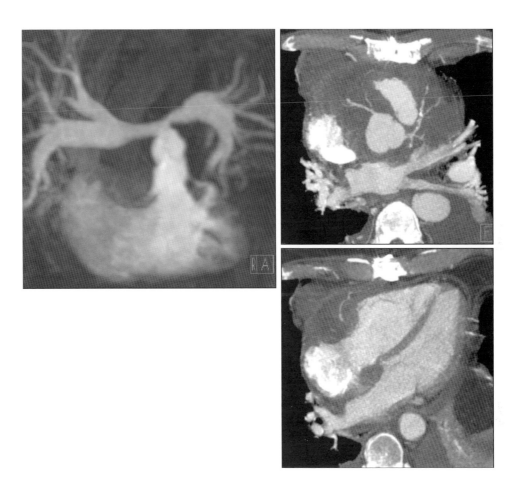

Figure 191 Mesothelioma

Format: MIP, MRA

These images show a soft tissue mass which encases the aorta and central pulmonary arteries. The narrowing of the central pulmonary arteries is shown in the magnetic resonance angiogram (MRA) (left upper panel). There was encasement and narrowing of the left superior pulmonary vein. The tumor mass surrounds the aortic root and extends along the interatrial septum. It also involves the right atrial wall and the inflow portion of the right ventricle with suspected myocardial invasion. It also extends through the pericardium in the area of the right atrioventricular groove, creating a separate paracardiac mass lesion of the right cardiophrenic angle, with complete encasement of the dominant RCA.

Pathology was consistent with a malignant spindle-cell neoplasm, in turn consistent with sarcomatoid mesothelioma.

CHAPTER 4.1.5, REFERENCES 169, 170

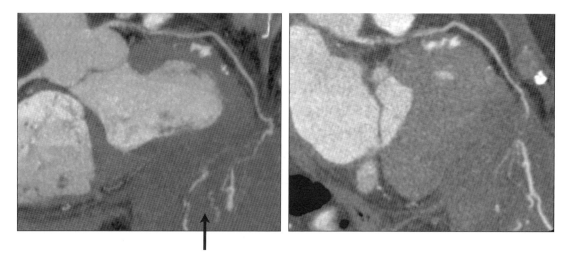

Figure 192   Pericardial sarcoma

Format: MPR, MIP

The identification of tumor vessels, as a sign of malignancy, is often possible secondary to the high spatial resolution of MDCT. This figure shows images of a large pericardial synovial sarcoma at the inferior aspect of the heart. The CT demonstrated tumor vessels (arrow).

CHAPTER 4.1.5, REFERENCES 169, 170

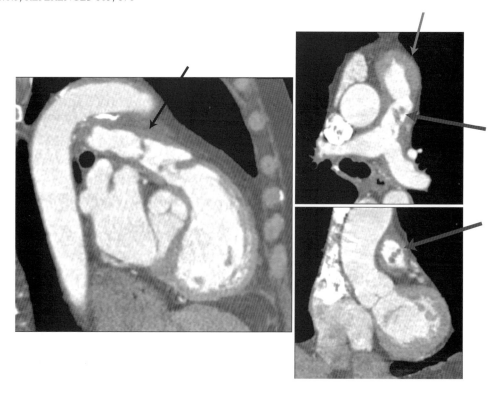

Figure 193   Neoplastic involvement of pulmonary artery

Format: MPR

This figure shows images from a patient with chest discomfort and worsening shortness of breath. The pericardium is normal. The pulmonary valve demonstrates a nodular appearance. There are mobile nodular lesions of the main pulmonary arteries (thick arrows). The walls of the pulmonary arteries are markedly thickened confluent with the abnormal increase of tissue of the mediastinum (thin arrows).

Additional lung lesions were observed. A malignant process was suspected.

CHAPTER 4.1.5, REFERENCES 169, 170

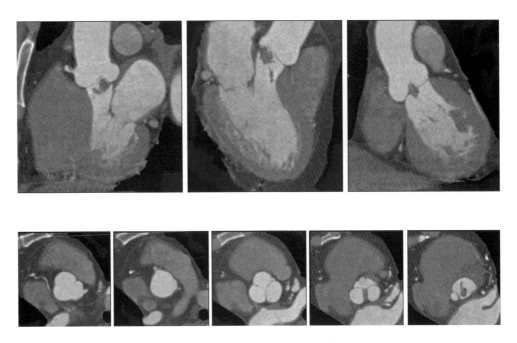

Figure 194   Aortic valve vegetation (1.1)

Format: MPR

This figure shows images of a patient with suspected endocarditis. An initial echocardiogram demonstrated a large mobile mass attached to the non-coronary cusp of the aortic valve, prolapsing into the left ventricular outflow tract (LVOT). The findings were consistent with vegetation or thrombus. There was associated moderate aortic regurgitation.

The CT scan was performed to assess coronary anatomy before surgery. Conventional cardiac catheterization was avoided because of the high risk for embolization. The CT images confirmed the soft tissue mass at the commissure between the non-coronary and left coronary cusps of the aortic valve.

The patient underwent open heart surgery with removal of the aortic valve thrombus/vegetation, repair of the aortic valve and coronary artery bypass. Intraoperatively, a large, friable mass originating at the commissure between the non- and left coronary cusps was found. The mass was adherent to the underside of the valve and commissure, but there was no invasion or damage of the valve leaflets. Pathologic examination was consistent with a thrombus or vegetation. Micro-organisms were not identified.

CHAPTER 4.1.6, REFERENCES 65, 171

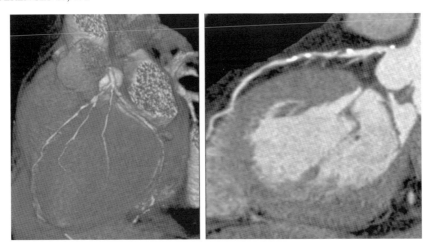

Figure 195   Aortic valve vegetation (1.2) (see also color section on p. 15)

Format: MPR

CT angiography demonstrated significant atherosclerotic disease of all three coronary arteries. In the proximal LAD, calcified and non-calcified atherosclerotic plaque was demonstrated, which was associated with > 50% stenosis.

CHAPTER 4.1.6, REFERENCES 65, 171

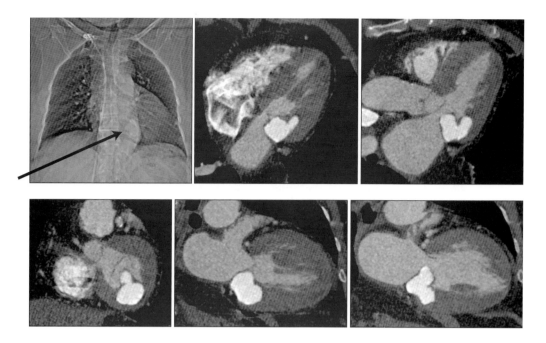

Figure 196 Severe mitral annular calcification

Format: MPR, X-ray

This figure shows images of a patient who was found to have an echogenic mass-like lesion in the area of the mitral annulus. The CT shows a well-circumscribed lobulated high-attenuation lesion, which appears to arise within the posterior mitral annulus and extends into the posterior left ventricular wall. The lesion measures approximately 3.3 × 3.2 × 2.7 cm. The attenuation value of the lesion is higher than that of the contrast-enhanced myocardial chambers, most consistent with calcium. The lesion demonstrates dense peripheral calcification. There is no evidence of feeding or draining vessels. The lesion is also identified on the CT topogram (arrow).

The findings are most consistent with mitral annular calcification.

CHAPTER 4.1.6, REFERENCES 65

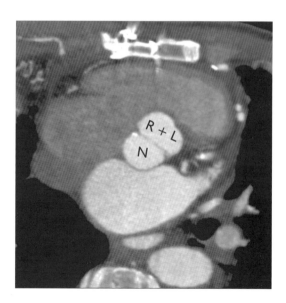

Figure 197 Bicuspid aortic valve (1)

Format: MPR

In contrast to a normal tricuspid aortic valve (Figure 40) this figure shows a bicuspid aortic valve. There is fusion of the left (L) and right (R) coronary cusps. The identification of the non-coronary cusp (N) is facilitated by its location between the left and right atria in the short-axis view.

CHAPTER 4.1.6, REFERENCES 65

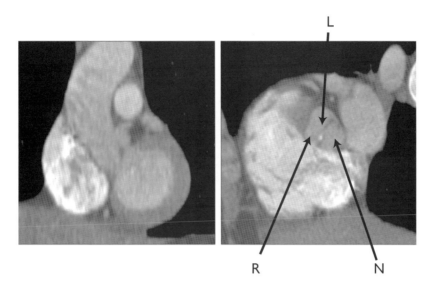

Figure 198 Bicuspid aortic valve (2)

Format: MPR

This figure shows images from a patient with aortic stenosis. The aortic valve is bicuspid, with congenital fusion of the left and right cusps (arrows). There is mild calcification of the aortic valve leaflets.

CHAPTER 4.1.6, REFERENCES 65

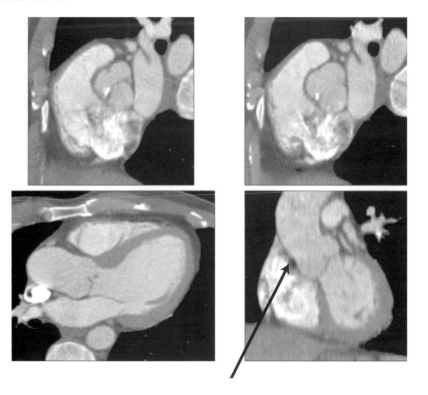

Figure 199 Bicuspid aortic valve with prominence of aortic root (3)

Format: MPR

Another example of a bicuspid valve is shown in this figure. There is fusion of the left and right coronary cusps and calcification of the commissure between the right and non-coronary cusps. There is asymmetric prominence of the non-coronary cusp. The aortic root is prominent and measures 4.3 cm. The sinotubular junction is maintained (arrow) and measures 3.5 cm. The mid-ascending thoracic aorta is prominent, measuring 4.5 cm.

CHAPTER 4.1.6, REFERENCES 65

173

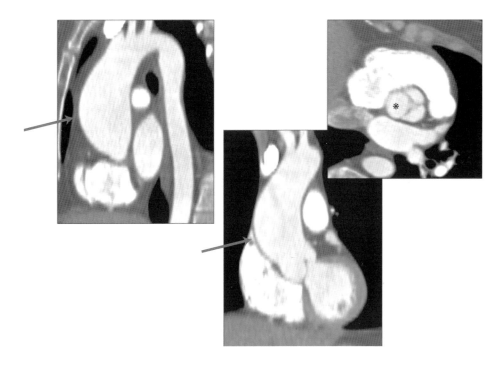

Figure 200 Bicuspid aortic valve (4)

Format: MIP

This figure shows a bicuspid aortic valve with partial fusion of left and right coronary cusps and asymmetric prominence of the non-coronary cusp (*). There is mild aneurysmal dilatation of the ascending aorta (arrows).

CHAPTER 4.1.6, REFERENCES 65, 171

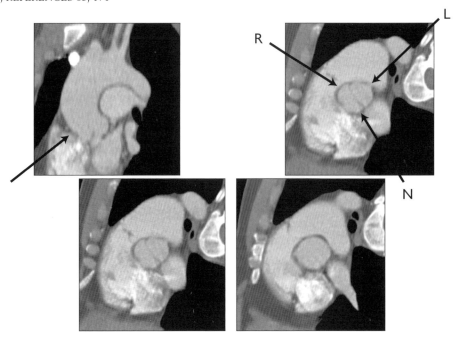

Figure 201 Bicuspid aortic valve (5)

Format: MIP

This figure shows a bicuspid aortic valve with fusion of the non-coronary (N) and right coronary (R) cusps (arrows, right upper panel). L, left coronary cusp. There is mild dilatation of the ascending aorta with a maximum diameter of 4.8 cm. There is mild-to-moderate effacement of the sinotubular junction (arrow, left upper panel).

CHAPTER 4.1.6, REFERENCES 65, 171

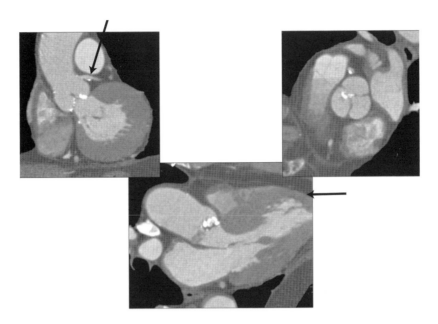

Figure 202 Aortic valve calcification in aortic stenosis

Format: MIP

CT can precisely describe the extent and location of valvular calcification. This figure shows calcification of the aortic valve leaflets in a patient with aortic stenosis. The aortic valve is trileaflet with severe calcification of the aortic valve leaflets. Also seen are calcified atherosclerotic, non-obstructive changes of the left main coronary artery (arrow, left upper panel) and mild left ventricular hypertrophy. There is a small area of myocardial thinning in the mid-to-apical LAD distribution consistent with subendocardial scarring (arrow, lower panel).

CHAPTER 4.1.6, REFERENCES 65, 171

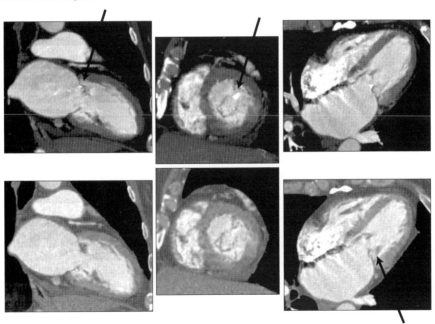

Figure 203 Mitral valve calcification in mitral stenosis

Format: MPR, MIP

Thickening and calcification of the mitral valve leaflets is associated with mitral stenosis. This figure shows images of a patient with chronic atrial fibrillation and mitral stenosis. The left atrial body shows moderate-to-severe dilatation without evidence of clot. There is thickening and calcification (arrows) of the mitral valve leaflets compatible with mitral stenosis.

CHAPTER 4.1.6, REFERENCES 65

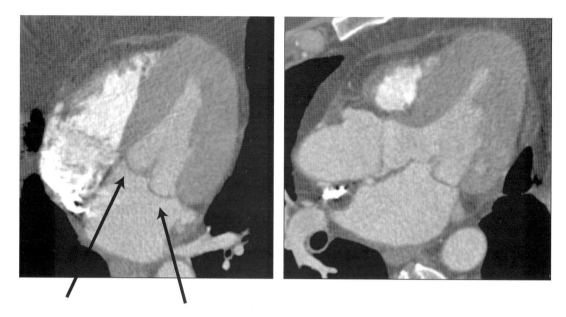

Figure 204   Mitral valve prolapse

Format: MIP

The images show mild thickening of the mitral valve leaflets. There is prolapse of both leaflets during systole, with bulging towards the left atrium (arrows). There is concentric left ventricular hypertrophy involving the left ventricle mid- and apical portions but sparing the left ventricular outflow tract.

CHAPTER 4.1.6, REFERENCES 65

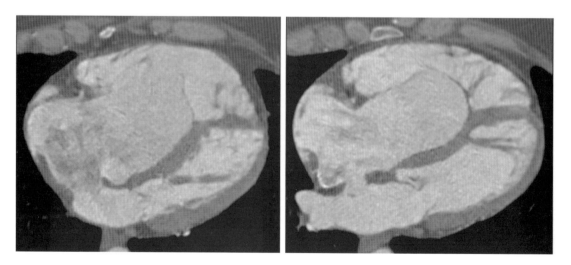

Figure 205   Ebstein's anomaly

Format: MPR

Ebstein's anomaly describes the displacement of the tricuspid valve towards the right ventricle.
The images show moderated dilatation of the right ventricle and severe dilatation of the right atrium. There is displacement of the septal component of the tricuspid valve from the normal position at the atrioventricular septum towards the right ventricle, consistent with changes of Ebstein's anomaly.

CHAPTER 4.1.6, REFERENCES 65

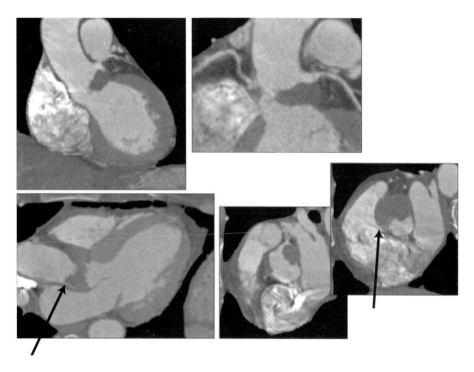

Figure 206   Aortic root mass (1.1)

Format: MIP

This figure shows an irregular mass involving the right and left coronary sinuses (arrows). While the mass approaches the coronary ostia, the coronary arteries are patent and there is no evidence of obstruction. The aortic valve leaflets are poorly visualized due to the presence of the soft tissue mass.

CHAPTER 4.1.6, REFERENCES 65, 171

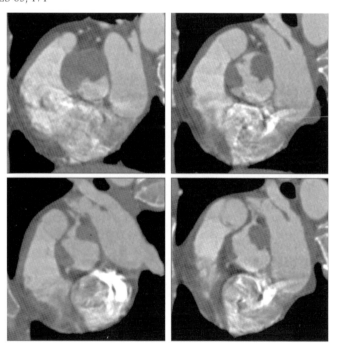

Figure 207   Aortic root mass (1.2)

Format: MIP

The relationship of the soft tissue mass to the sinuses of Valsalva and the coronary arteries is shown in these short-axis views.

CHAPTER 4.1.6, REFERENCES 65, 171

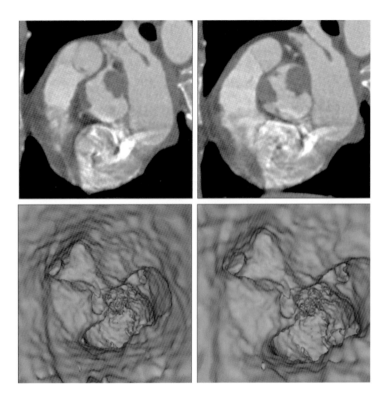

Figure 208   Aortic root mass (1.3) (see also color section on p. 16)

Format: MPR, VRI

This figure shows MPR and volume-rendered images of the mass. The VRIs give an endoscopic view inside the vessel lumen (lower panels).

CHAPTER 4.1.6, REFERENCES 65, 171

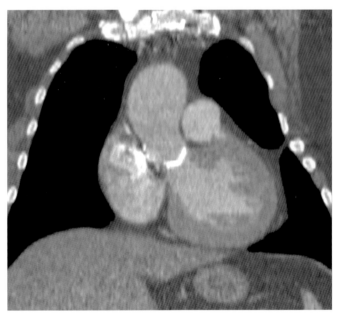

Figure 209   Aortic valve replacement with mechanical valve (1)

Format: MPR

This figure shows a low-profile mechanical prosthesis in the aortic position. The root measures 3.0 cm. The sinotubular junction is intact. It is followed by fusiform dilatation of the mid-ascending aorta, measuring 5.3 cm.

CHAPTER 4.1.6, REFERENCES 65, 171

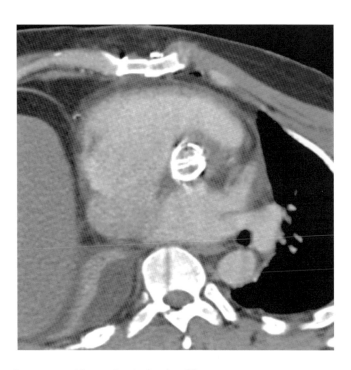

Figure 210 Aortic valve replacement with mechanical valve (2)

Format: MPR

A short-axis view at the aortic root shows a mechanical valve (St Jude) in the aortic valve position. The systolic image shows the open tilting disks of the valve.

CHAPTER 4.1.6, REFERENCES 65, 171

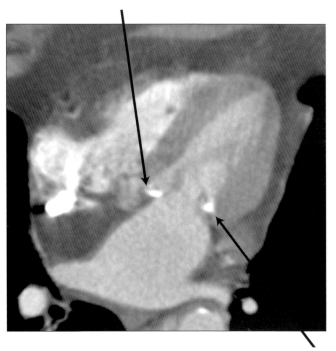

Figure 211 Mitral valve repair with prosthetic ring

Format: MIP

This figure shows an image of a patient after mitral valve repair. A prosthetic annular ring is seen in the mitral annular position (arrows). In addition, lipomatous septal hypertrophy is seen (Chapter 4.1.1.5).

CHAPTER 4.1.6, REFERENCES 65

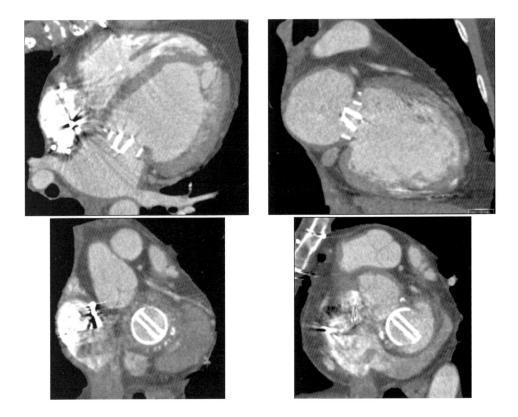

Figure 212   Mitral valve replacement with mechanical valve

Format: MPR

This figure shows an image of a patient after mitral valve replacement. The cardiac chambers show mild dilatation of the left ventricle. There is replacement of the mitral valve with a mechanical prosthesis. The tilting disks are well seen.

CHAPTER 4.1.6, REFERENCES 65

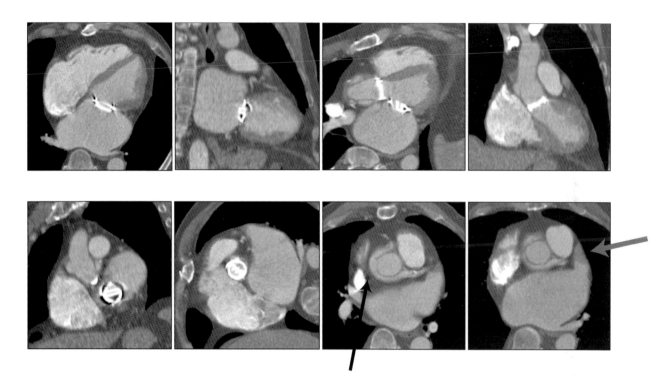

Figure 213   Mitral valve and aortic valve replacement

Format: MPR

This figure shows images of a patient after mitral and aortic valve replacement and coronary bypass surgery. The cardiac chambers are notable for severe left atrial dilatation and moderate right atrial dilatation. There is a filling defect in the left atrial appendage consistent with thrombus or slow flow (thick arrow, right lower panel). The left and right ventricles have normal dimensions. There is evidence of mitral valve replacement with a mechanical valve.

There is also evidence of a valved conduit graft of the ascending thoracic aorta, with a mechanical aortic valve. In the lateral segment of the grafted ascending aorta is an interposed graft dividing into two limbs, connecting to the native coronary arteries (black arrow). Beyond the graft of the ascending aorta, the native aorta has normal dimensions.

CHAPTER 4.1.6, REFERENCES 65

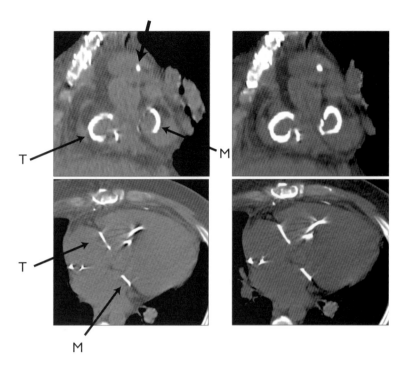

Figure 214 Mitral valve and tricuspid valve repair with prosthetic rings

Format: MPR, MIP

This figure shows non-contrast-enhanced images of a patient after mitral and tricuspid valve repair. Prosthetic rings are seen in the mitral (M) and tricuspid (T) position. A pulmonary artery catheter is seen extending into the central pulmonary artery (thick arrow).

CHAPTER 4.1.6, REFERENCES 65

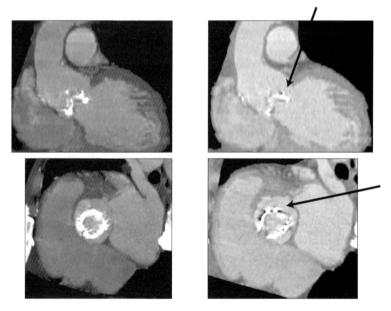

Figure 215 Aortic valve dehiscence

Format: MPR, MIP

This figure shows images of a patient with a remote aortic valve replacement and suspected endocarditis. There is a bioprosthetic Carpentier–Edwards aortic valve and supracoronary graft of the ascending aorta. There is increased size of the aortic root (5.2 cm) with separation of the valve ring at the left and right sinuses of Valsalva (arrows).
During surgery, an aortic periprosthetic leak was identified and replacement with a homograft performed.

CHAPTER 4.1.6, REFERENCES 65, 171

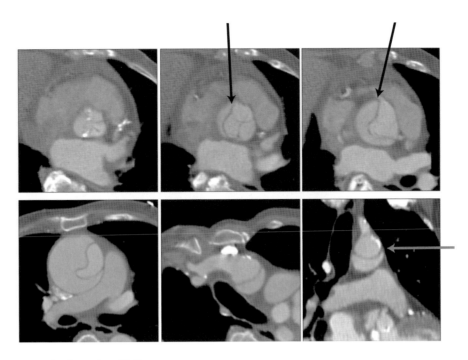

Figure 216   Type A aortic dissection (1.1)

Format: MIP

In the assessment of aortic dissections and intramural hematomas, an important aspect is the involvement of the ascending aorta. Type A dissections, which involve the ascending aorta, are typically corrected surgically as soon as possible.
The figure shows a type A dissection. The dissection flap (arrows) originates in the aortic root (upper panels) and extends throughout the ascending thoracic aorta and aortic arch (lower panel). In the dilated mid-ascending aorta (lower left panel) the smaller true lumen is surrounded by the larger false lumen.

CHAPTER 4.1.7, REFERENCES 172–176

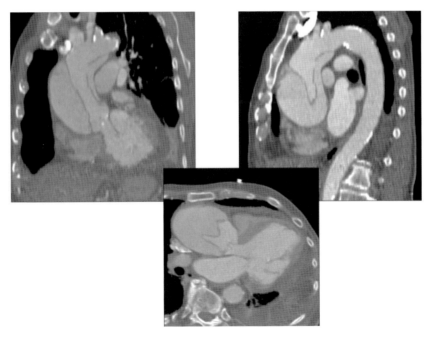

Figure 217   Type A aortic dissection (1.2)

Format: MPR, MIP

The corresponding sagittal reconstructions show the extent of the dissection in the ascending aorta and aortic arch.

CHAPTER 4.1.7, REFERENCES 172–176

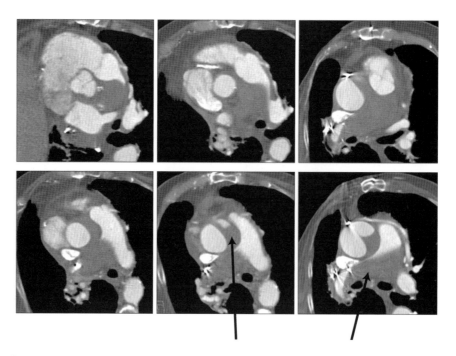

Figure 218 Type A aortic dissection with hemopericardium (2.1)

Format: MPR

The identification of acute complications, in particular rupture, hemoperitoneum and hemopericardium, is crucial in the clinical assessment of patients with acute dissection.

The images in this figure show an acute type A aortic dissection beginning at the sinotubular junction and extending into the arch. The false channel is partially thrombosed (arrow, lower middle panel). There is a hemorrhagic pericardial effusion, which compresses the right pulmonary artery (arrow, lower right panel).

CHAPTER 4.1.7, REFERENCES 172–176

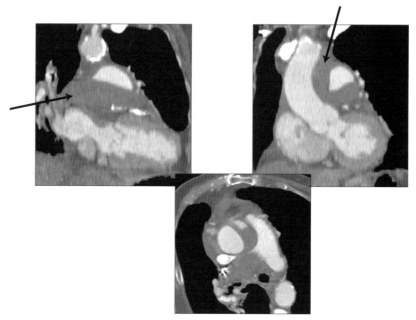

Figure 219 Type A aortic dissection with hemopericardium (2.2)

Format: MPR

A hemopericardium at the superior aspect of the left ventricle, causing compression of the pulmonary artery, is shown in this figure (arrows).

CHAPTER 4.1.7, REFERENCES 172–176

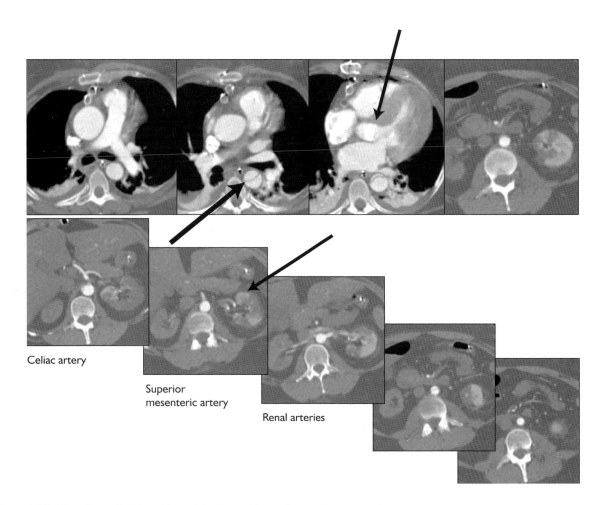

Celiac artery

Superior
mesenteric artery

Renal arteries

Figure 220 Type B aortic dissection with visceral branch vessel compression

Format: MPR

This figure shows images from a patient with recent aortic valve replacement and acute postoperative clinical deterioration with loss of peripheral pulses. There was suspicion for an aortic dissection. The CT scan shows evidence of aortic valve replacement with a mechanical valve (thin arrow, upper panels). There is no evidence of dissection of the ascending thoracic aorta and aortic arch with patent aortic arch branch vessels.

There is evidence of a type B aortic dissection beginning in the mid-descending thoracic aorta (thick arrow) and extending into the infrarenal abdominal aorta, ending above the origin of the inferior mesenteric artery. There is almost complete compression of the true lumen in the lower descending thoracic and abdominal aorta involving the origins of the celiac artery, superior mesenteric artery and right renal artery, which originate from the true lumen. The left renal artery originates from the false lumen.

There is severe hypoperfusion of both kidneys, which is uniform on the right and patchy on the left (thin arrow, upper panels). There is no evidence of pneumatosis or bowel wall thickening to suggest mesenteric ischemia.

The patient underwent emergency endovascular repair with placement of two sequential stent grafts in the proximal and mid-descending thoracic aorta.

CHAPTER 4.1.7, REFERENCES 172–176

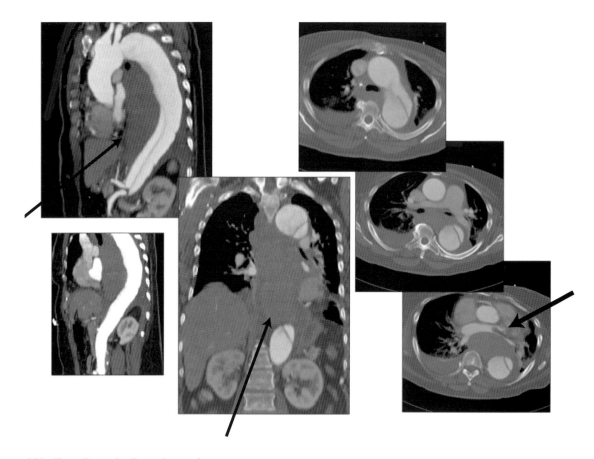

Figure 221 Type B aortic dissection and rupture

Format: MIP

This figure shows images of a patient with a type B aortic dissection beginning just beyond the origin of the left subclavian artery. The dissection extends throughout the thoracic and abdominal aorta. There are luminal irregularities in the aortic isthmus, which may represent the site of rupture. The mediastinum is notable for a large amount of blood products surrounding the descending thoracic aorta, extending to the level of the diaphragm (thin arrows). This leads to partial compression of the left atrium and pulmonary veins (thick arrow). There are bilateral pleural effusions with increased density, consistent with complex and hemorrhagic effusions.

CHAPTER 4.1.7, REFERENCES 172–176

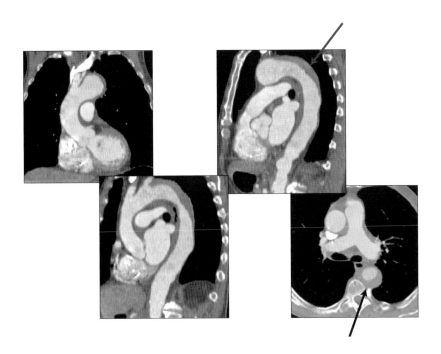

Figure 222 Intramural hematoma (1)

Format: MPR, MIP

Because of the superior image detail (high spatial resolution), CT scanners allow reliable assessment of the vessel wall. CT is therefore well suited for the identification of intramural hematomas.
This figure shows an intramural hematoma of the descending thoracic aorta. There is wall thickening of the isthmus and descending thoracic aorta (arrow, right upper panel). The cross-sectional image shows the crescent shape of the intramural hematoma in the mid-descending aorta (arrow, right lower panel).

CHAPTER 4.1.7, REFERENCES 172–178

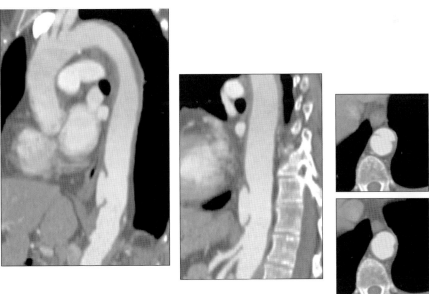

Figure 223 Intramural hematoma (2)

Format: MPR

This figure shows a chronic intramural hematoma of the descending thoracic aorta. Wall thickening of the isthmus and upper descending thoracic aorta is consistent with residuals of an intramural hematoma. In the descending thoracic aorta there is an area of intimal disruption associated with mild bulging of the aorta (3.9 cm).

CHAPTER 4.1.7, REFERENCES 172–178

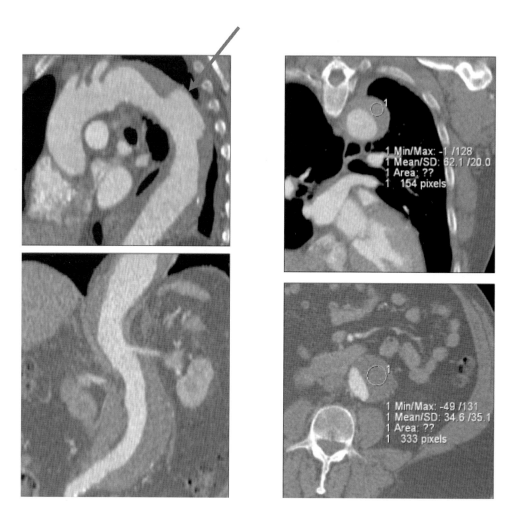

Figure 224 Intramural hematoma and abdominal aneurysm

Format: MPR

This figure shows an intramural hematoma of the descending thoracic aorta with enlargement of the involved aortic segments (upper panels). The maximum diameter in the retrocardiac descending aorta is 6.3 cm. There is a large area of communication between the lumen and the hematoma in the proximal descending aorta (arrow). The intramural hematoma ends in the suprarenal aorta.

There is an additional infrarenal abdominal aortic aneurysm with maximum diameter of 5.1 cm (lower panels). The difference in Hounsfield units helps to differentiate the two entities.

CHAPTER 4.1.7, REFERENCES 172–178

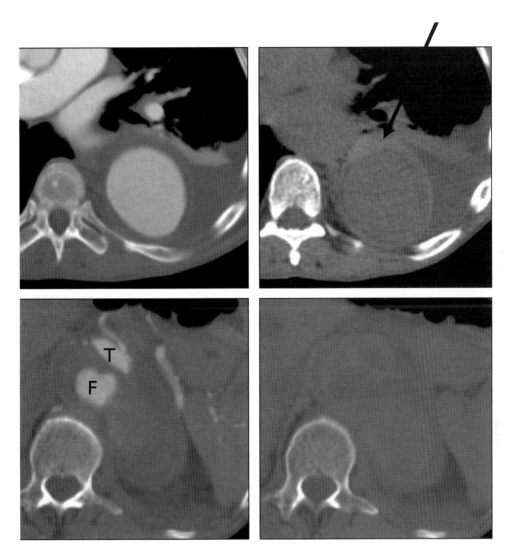

Figure 225   Intramural hematoma: increased vessel wall opacity

Format: MPR

This figure demonstrates aortic wall enhancement secondary to an acute/subacute intramural hematoma. This becomes obvious by comparison of the contrast-enhanced (left panels) and non-contrast-enhanced images (right panels). In the descending thoracic aorta, there is inhomogeneous radio-opacity of the thickened aortic wall consistent with an acute intramural hematoma (arrow, upper panels). The aorta further dilates at the level above the diaphragm where a true (T) and false (F) lumen of the dissection process can be differentiated (lower panels).

CHAPTER 4.1.7, REFERENCES 172–178

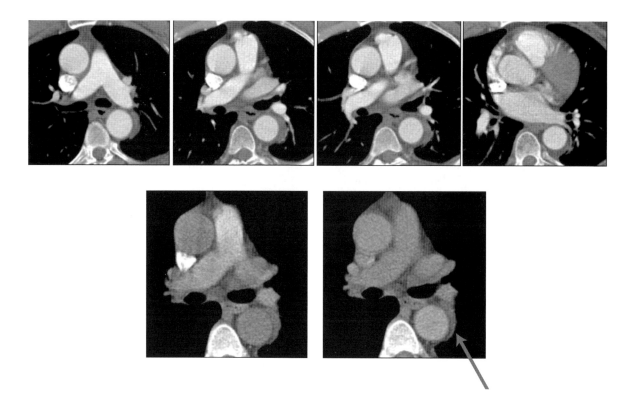

Figure 226   Intramural hematoma: differential diagnosis

Format: MPR

This figure shows a small atelectasis of the lung adjacent to the descending thoracic aorta (arrow), which mimics the crescent appearance of an intramural hematoma. The upper panels show different axial slices at the level around the bifurcation of the pulmonary arteries. The lower images show views during injection of the contrast bolus.

CHAPTER 4.1.7, REFERENCES 172–178

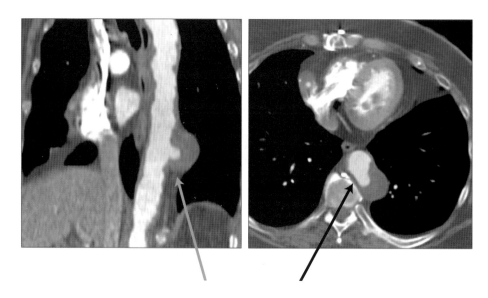

Figure 227   Penetrating ulceration

Format: MPR

Other findings seen in acute and chronic settings are large penetrating ulcerations. This figure shows a focal penetrating ulceration in the retrocardiac descending thoracic aorta measuring 3.0 × 5.6 cm (arrows).

CHAPTER 4.1.7, REFERENCES 172–179

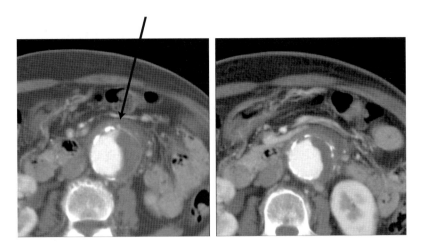

Figure 228   Leaking abdominal aneurysm

Format: MPR

This figure shows axial images of an infrarenal aortic aneurysm. The ill-defined luminal border and contrast enhancement surrounding the aneurysm are consistent with chronic leakage (arrow).

CHAPTER 4.1.7, REFERENCES 172–178

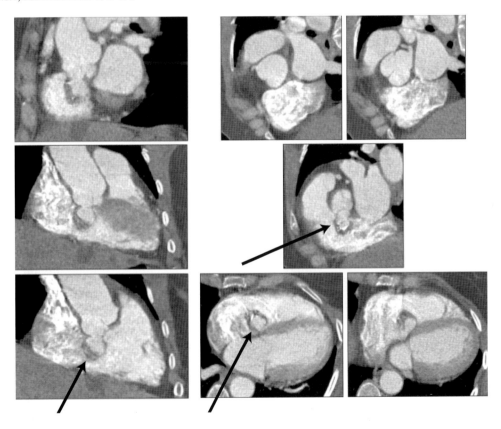

Figure 229   Sinus of Valsalva aneurysm (1)

Format: MPR

CT is routinely performed for the identification of thoracic and abdominal aortic aneurysms. A strength of CT is the ability to reconstruct images perpendicular to the vessel axis for each segment of the aorta.

An example of a sinus Valsalva aneurysm is shown in this figure (arrows). It originates from the non-coronary cusp and measures 2.5 × 2.1 cm. It is in close relation to the atrial aspect of the septal leaflet of the tricuspid valve. The aneurysm is partially thrombosed but well perfused in the central portion. No communication is evident (Movies 39–41).

CHAPTER 4.1.7, REFERENCES 172, 173

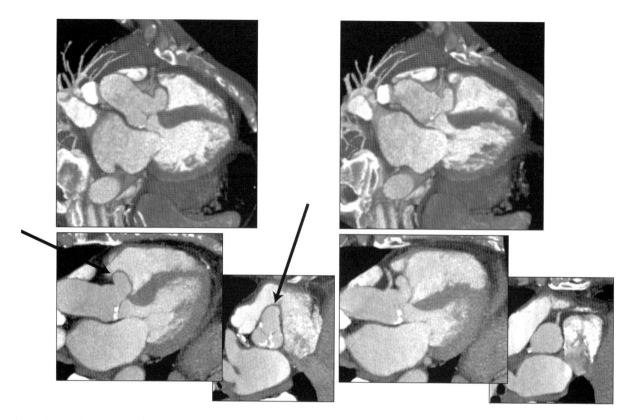

Figure 230   Sinus of Valsalva aneurysm (2)

Format: MIP, VRI

Another example of a sinus of Valsalva aneurysm is shown in this figure. There is a saccular outpouching of the right coronary sinus limited to its lower portion, immediately above the trileaflet aortic valve (arrows). This saccular outpouching measures approximately 1.4 × 2.4 × 1.9 cm. The RCA arises from the more superior portion of the otherwise normal-appearing right coronary sinus of Valsalva.

The findings are consistent with a sinus of Valsalva aneurysm of the right coronary cusp.

CHAPTER 4.1.7, REFERENCES 172, 173

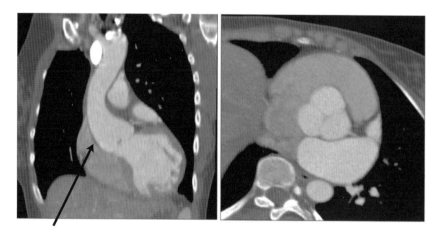

Figure 231   Dilated aortic root

Format: MIP

This figure shows images of a patient with Marfan's syndrome. The aortic valve is trileaflet. There is a dilated aortic root with moderate effacement of the sinotubular junction (arrow). Beyond the dilated root, the aorta has normal dimensions. The pattern of dilatation is consistent with annulo-aortic ectasia.

CHAPTER 4.1.7, REFERENCES 172, 173

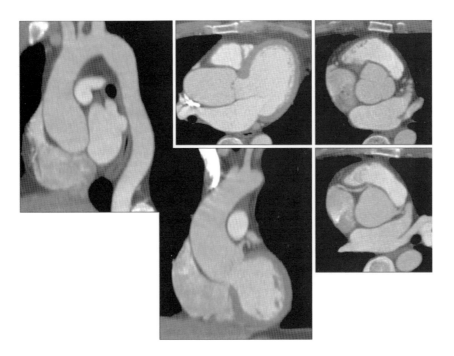

Figure 232 Annulo-aortic ectasia

Format: MPR

Another example of annulo-aortic ectasia with prominence of the aortic root and proximal ascending aorta (maximum diameter 5.2 cm) is shown. There is associated moderate effacement of the sinotubular junction.

CHAPTER 4.1.7, REFERENCES 172, 173

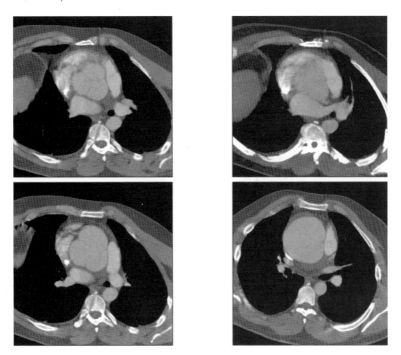

Figure 233   Ascending aortic aneurysm: Marfan's syndrome (1.1)

Format: MPR

This figure shows axial images of an aneurysm of the aortic root and ascending aorta in a patient with Marfan's syndrome. There is massive dilatation of the aortic root, measuring 8 cm in diameter.

CHAPTER 4.1.7, REFERENCES 172, 173

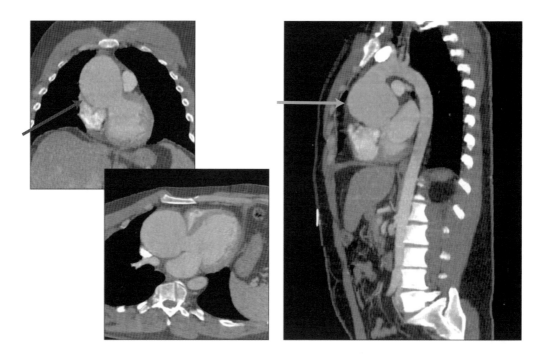

Figure 234   Ascending aortic aneurysm: Marfan's syndrome (1.2)

Format: MIP

The massive aneurysm of the aortic root and ascending aorta is demonstrated in these oblique images (arrows).

CHAPTER 4.1.7, REFERENCES 172, 173

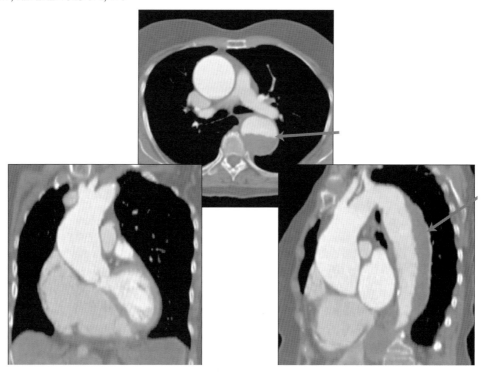

Figure 235   Descending aortic aneurysm

Format: MPR

This figure shows an aortic aneurysm of the descending thoracic aorta, with a moderate-to-severe amount of adherent wall thrombus (arrows). There is also dilatation of the ascending aorta.

CHAPTER 4.1.7, REFERENCES 172, 173

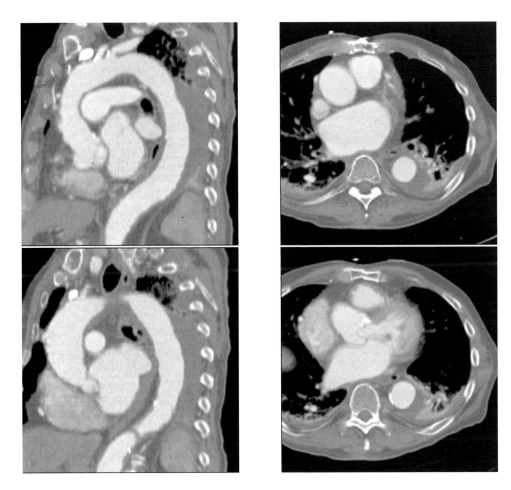

Figure 236   Aneurysm: differential diagnosis

Format: MPR

This figure shows images of a patient with bilateral small-to-moderate pleural effusions. In the descending thoracic aorta the fluid lies adjacent to the aorta, and on some images has an appearance similar to an aneurysm or intramural hematoma (upper panels). However, close observation demonstrates that aortic wall and fluid are separate (lower panels).

CHAPTER 4.1.7, REFERENCES 172, 173

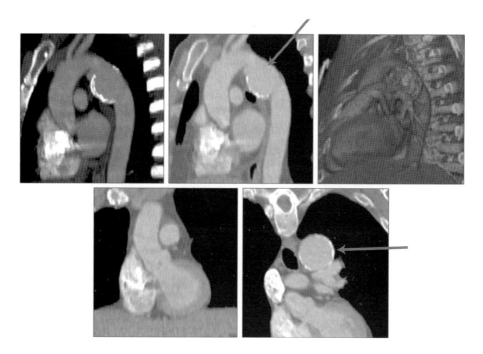

Figure 237   Post-traumatic aneurysm (see also color section on p. 16)

Format: MPR, MIP, VRI

This figure shows images of a patient with a remote history of a motor vehicle accident. There is a focal aneurysm in the area of the isthmus and proximal descending thoracic aorta, with eccentric expansion and calcification of its anterolateral surface (arrows). The maximum diameter is 4.8 cm. Proximal and distal to the aneurysm, the aorta has normal dimensions and minimal atherosclerotic changes.

CHAPTER 4.1.7, REFERENCES 172, 173

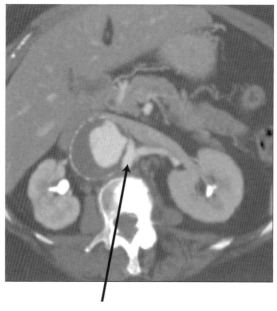

Figure 238   Dissection and aneurysm

Format: MPR

If an aortic dissection is superimposed on an existing aneurysm, the dissection typically ends proximal to or at the aneurysm. Only occasionally, the dissection extends beyond the area of the aneurysm.

An example is shown in this figure, where the false channel of the dissection extends beyond the infrarenal abdominal aortic aneurysm (arrow).

CHAPTER 4.1.7, REFERENCES 172, 173

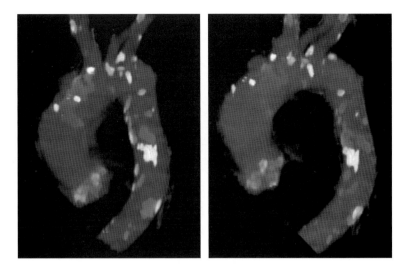

Figure 239   Calcified aorta

Format: VRI

An important application of CT is perioperative imaging of the aorta in patients undergoing cardiac and aortic surgery. In patients undergoing open heart surgery, the local extent of calcified atherosclerotic plaque can determine the cannulation site for cardiopulmonary bypass. To assess the amount of calcification, a non-contrast-enhanced CT scan is performed.
In this figure, volume-rendered images from a patient with severe calcification of the aorta and aortic valve are shown. The soft tissues are faded, allowing a three-dimensional image of the calcification.

CHAPTER 4.1.7, REFERENCES 172, 173

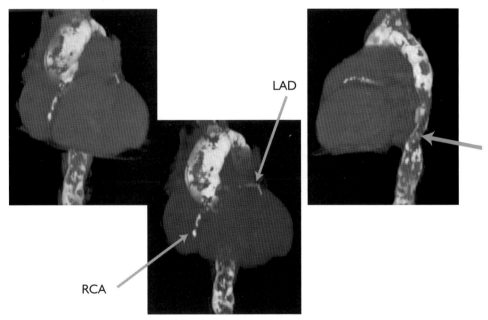

Figure 240   Calcified aorta in patient with history of aortitis

Format: VRI

This figure shows images of a severely calcified aorta in a patient with a remote history of Takayasu's aortitis. The patient now presented with left main coronary artery stenosis.
The CT images show severe circumferential calcification of the thoracic aorta with an area of narrowing in the descending thoracic aorta (thick arrow). The calcified right coronary artery (RCA) and left anterior descending coronary artery (LAD) are seen (thin arrows).
Because of the severe aortic calcification, the patient was not considered to be a candidate for open heart surgery and subsequently underwent left main percutaneous coronary intervention (PCI).

CHAPTER 4.1.7, REFERENCES 172, 173

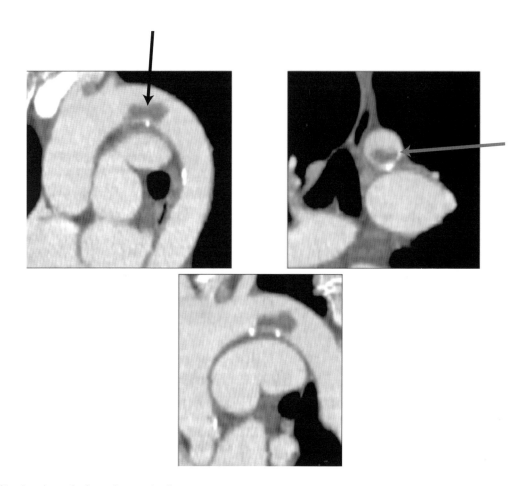

Figure 241   Aortic arch thrombus and atheroma

Format: MPR

Contrast-enhanced scans can assess the amount of calcified and non-calcified atherosclerotic plaque, which appears to be related to postoperative stroke incidence.

This figure shows a protruding soft tissue in the aortic arch, consistent with thrombus (arrows). There is underlying calcified atherosclerotic plaque.

CHAPTER 4.1.7, REFERENCES 172, 173, 180, 181

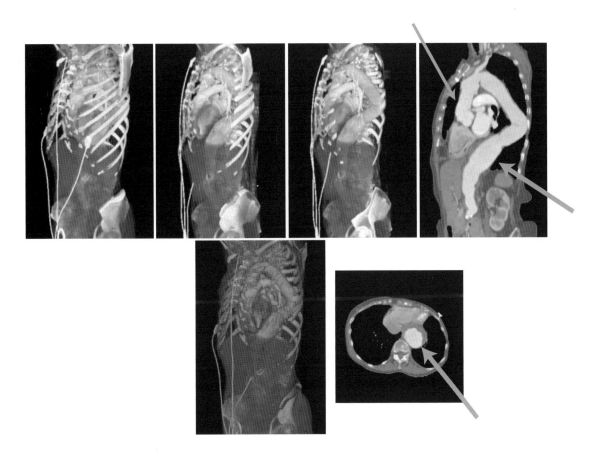

Figure 242 Preoperative assessment of thoracoabdominal aortic aneurysm (see also color section on p. 17)

Format: MPR, VRI

Preoperative CT can help in deciding about the surgical access site in patients with thoracoabdominal aneurysms.
This is demonstrated in this figure. There is evidence of a supracoronary graft of the ascending thoracic aorta, which is intact
(thin arrow). Beyond the graft, there is mild dilatation of the arch measuring 4.7 cm in the proximal segment, and 2.3 cm
in the distal segment. There is mild ectasia of the isthmus measuring 3.8 cm and mid-descending thoracic aorta measuring
3.9 cm. There is a thoracoabdominal aneurysm with a maximum diameter of 7.4 × 6.0 cm in the retrocardiac descending
thoracic aorta (thick arrows). There is a moderate amount of adherent wall thrombus (right lower panel). The aorta then
tapers to 3.7 cm at the diaphragm and 3.3 cm in the suprarenal segment. There is no evidence of dissection. The VRIs show
the ribs and the aneurysm and allow planning of the surgical access site.

CHAPTER 4.1.7, REFERENCES 172

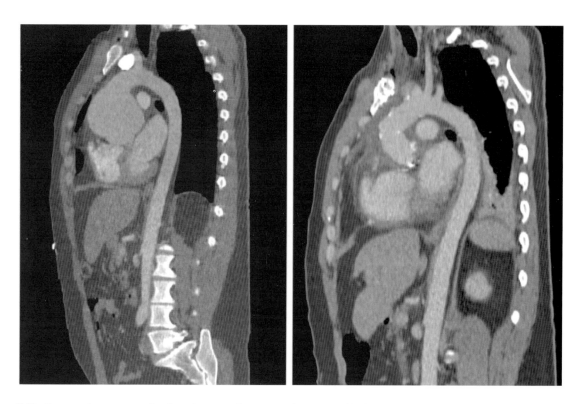

Figure 243   Pre- and postoperative imaging: aortic root replacement (1.1)

Format: MIP

Postoperative CT scans are useful in the assessment of surgical results.

This figure shows pre- and post-operative images of an aneurysm of the ascending aorta. This patient with Marfan's syndrome presented with severe dilatation of the ascending aorta (left panel). The postoperative CT demonstrates replacement of the aortic valve, and sequential grafts covering the aortic root, ascending aorta and parts of the aortic arch (right panel).

CHAPTER 4.1.7, REFERENCES 172, 173

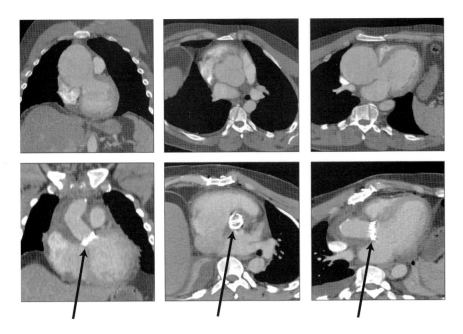

Figure 244   Pre- and postoperative imaging: aortic root replacement (1.2)

Format: MIP

These images show the aortic valve, aortic root and ascending aorta before (upper panels) and after (lower panels) surgery. A mechanical aortic valve prosthesis (arrows) is placed inside a graft of the root and ascending aorta (composite graft). The coronary arteries are reimplanted into the graft.

CHAPTER 4.1.7, REFERENCES 172, 173

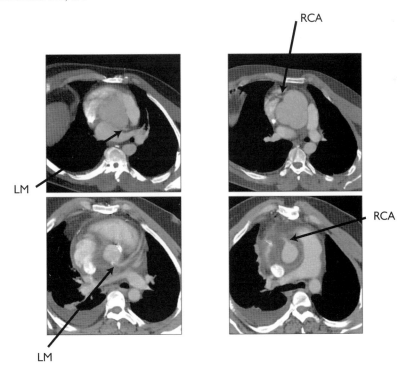

Figure 245   Pre- and postoperative imaging: aortic root replacement (1.3)

Format: MIP

The origin of the coronary arteries from the dilated root preoperatively (upper panels) and reimplanted coronary arteries from the graft after surgery (lower panels) are shown. RCA, right coronary artery; LM, left main coronary artery.

CHAPTER 4.1.7, REFERENCES 172, 173

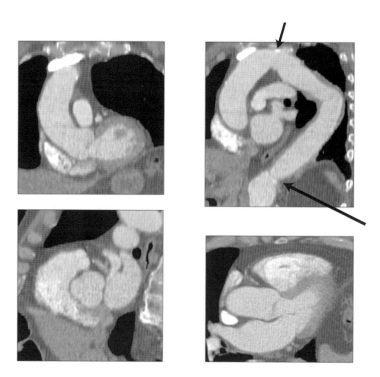

Figure 246   Surgical grafts: postoperative

Format: MPR

This figure shows images of a surgical graft of the upper descending thoracic aorta. The graft is intact and the proximal and distal anastomoses are seen (arrows).

CHAPTER 4.1.7, REFERENCES 172, 173

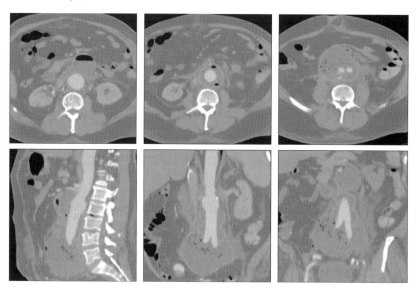

Figure 247   Infected abdominal aortic aneurysm (AAA) graft

Format: MPR

Postoperative CT scans are useful in the assessment of surgical results and complications. In the early postoperative phase, complications at the repair site or in the operative field, including mediastinal hematoma or infection, pericardial or pleural effusion and pneumothorax, can be identified.

This figure shows images of a patient several days after placement of an infrarenal aorto-bifemoral graft. There is a large perigraft fluid collection consistent with graft infection. The more superior fluid collection with a prominent air fluid level suggests the possibility of an aorto-enteric fistula as the source of the infection (left upper panel).

CHAPTER 4.1.7, REFERENCES 172, 173

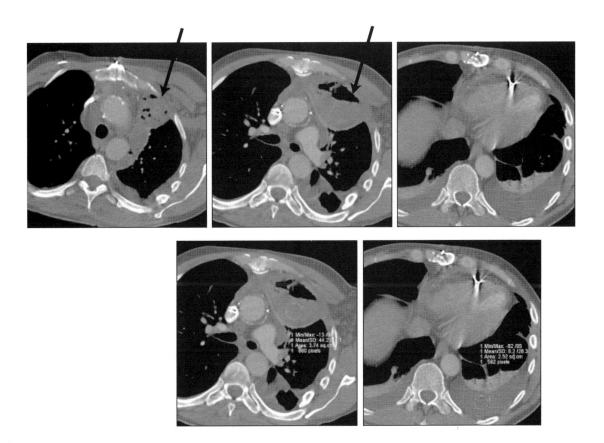

Figure 248 Postoperative empyema

Format: MPR

This figure shows images of a patient with a remote history of aortic valve replacement and recent bacterial endocarditis. Ten days before the CT scan the patient underwent replacement of the aortic valve and ascending thoracic aorta using a composite graft. The patient remained febrile and demonstrated an elevated white blood count.

The CT scan shows evidence of aortic valve replacement and replacement of the ascending thoracic aorta with a composite graft. The graft is surrounded by the expected postoperative blood products. There is a small-size right-sided and a moderate-size left-sided pleural effusion with adjacent atelectasis. There is a large air/fluid collection measuring 13 × 7 cm in the left upper pleural space, most consistent with an abscess (arrows). There are small mediastinal lymph nodes and prominent axillary lymph nodes.

CHAPTER 4.1.7, REFERENCES 172, 173

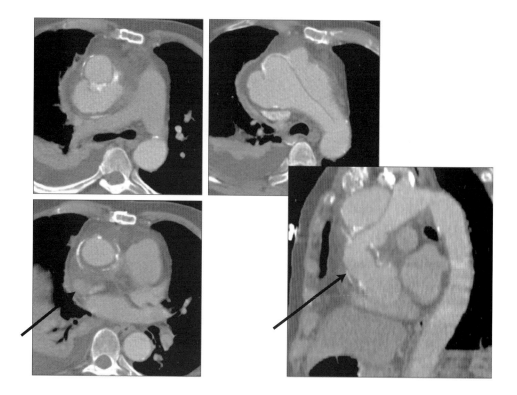

Figure 249   Endocarditis and ascending aortic graft infection

Format: MPR

This figure shows images of a patient with a remote history of aortic dissection and surgical grafting of the ascending aorta. The patient was evaluated for suspected endocarditis.

The CT scan shows a moderate-sized right pleural effusion with right lower lobe atelectasis and consolidation. The aortic root is dilated, measuring 5.6 cm. There has been replacement of the proximal ascending aorta with a supracoronary graft (arrow, right lower panel). There is fluid surrounding the graft, which compresses the superior vena cava (arrow, left lower panel). The appearance is suspicious for graft infection. Beyond the distal anatomy of the graft there is a dilated aortic arch with a dissection flap. The maximum diameter is 7.5 cm.

Findings during subsequent surgery were consistent with endocarditis of the native aortic valve caused by *Staphylococcus aureus*. The graft of the ascending aorta was surrounded by pus.

CHAPTER 4.1.7, REFERENCES 172, 173

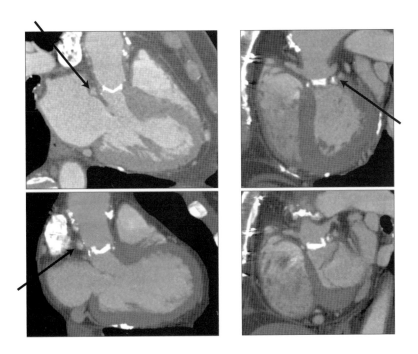

Figure 250 Root abscess (1.1)

Format: MPR, MIP

This figure shows images of a patient who presented with fever, months after aortic valve replacement with a mechanical valve. The small contrast-filled cavities at the aortic root are consistent with sequelae of a root abscess (arrows).

CHAPTER 4.1.7, REFERENCES 172, 173

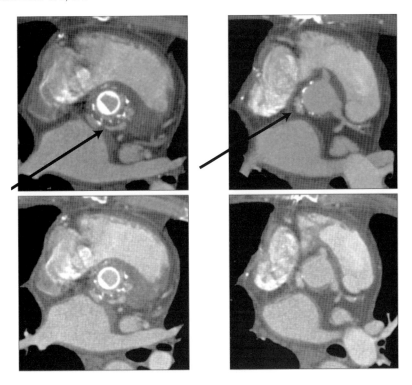

Figure 251 Root abscess (1.2)

Format: MPR, MIP

The small cavities are better appreciated in these cross-sectional images of the aortic root (arrows).

CHAPTER 4.1.7, REFERENCES 172, 173

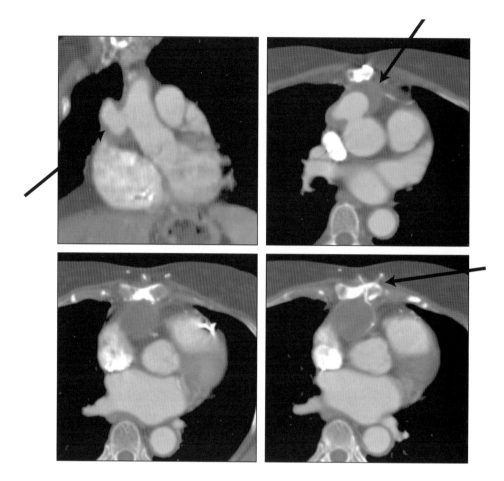

Figure 252 Mycotic pseudoaneurysm of the ascending aorta

Format: MIP

This figure shows images of a patient who developed a mycotic pseudoaneurysm after mitral valve repair. The sternum demonstrated osseous changes consistent with chronic osteomyelitis. Residuals of retained epicardial pacer wires are seen in the subcutaneous tissue of the anterior chest wall (arrow, right lower panel). There is a small amount of subcutaneous fluid surrounding it.

There is a presumably mycotic pseudoaneurysm arising from the mid-aorta, in a retrosternal location. The saccular outpouching (not including the native aorta) measures 3.6 × 4.7 × 4.7 cm and is partially thrombus filled (arrows, upper panels).

CHAPTER 4.1.7, REFERENCES 172, 173

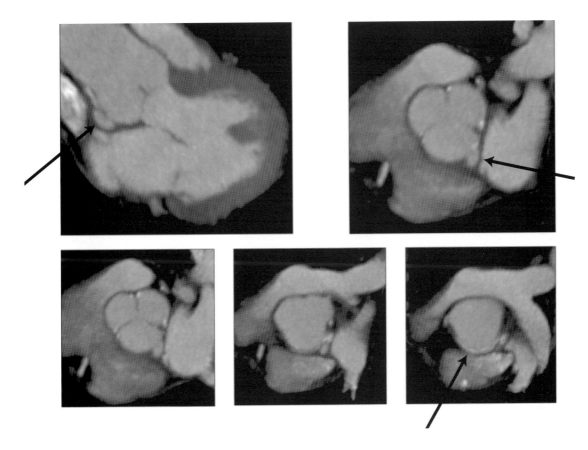

Figure 253   Postoperative pseudoaneurysm (1)

Format: MIP

This figure shows images of a patient with remote placement of a supracoronary graft of the aorta for type A aortic dissection repair.
There is a prominent native aortic root measuring 4.2 cm and a supracoronary graft of the ascending aorta. There is a small saccular outpouching at the proximal anastomosis adjacent to the non-coronary sinus of Valsalva, consistent with a pseudoaneurysm (arrows, upper panels). Suture material at the proximal anastomosis of the supracoronary graft of the ascending aorta is demonstrated (arrow, right lower panel).

CHAPTER 4.1.7, REFERENCES 172, 173

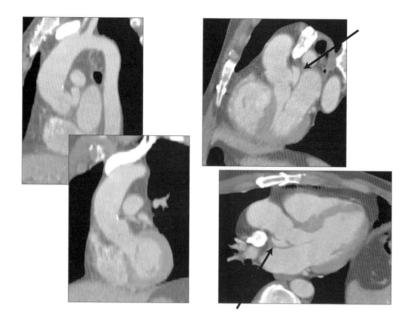

Figure 254   Postoperative pseudoaneurysm (2.1)

Format: MPR

This figure shows images of a patient with a history of aortic valve endocarditis and subsequent homograft replacement of the aortic root with reimplantation of the coronary arteries.

The CT images show a pseudoaneurysm originating primarily from the posterior aspect of the left coronary cusp (arrows). The cavity measures 2.3 × 0.8 cm. The pseudoaneurysm extends superiorly as well as inferiorly into the area of fibrous confluence of the anterior mitral leaflet and the posterior wall of the aorta.

CHAPTER 4.1.7, REFERENCES 172, 173

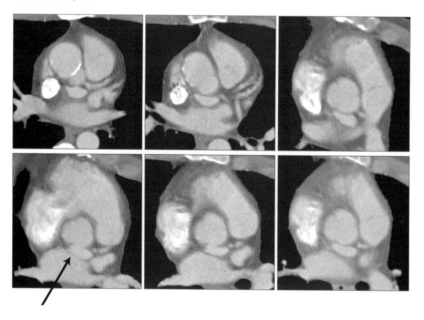

Figure 255   Title: postoperative pseudoaneurysm (2.2)

Format: MPR

Axial images at the aortic root demonstrate the origin of the pseudoaneurysm from the posterior aspect of the left coronary cusp, straddling the commissure between the left and non-coronary cusps (arrow, left lower panel).

During subsequent open heart surgery, an autologous pericardial patch repair of the opening to the subvalvular space was performed. Additionally, an aortic valve replacement was performed using a Carpentier–Edwards valve.

CHAPTER 4.1.7, REFERENCES 172, 173

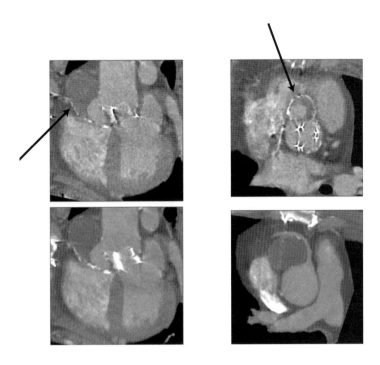

Figure 256   Postoperative pseudoaneurysm (3)

Format: MPR, MIP

This figure shows images of a patient with a remote aortic valve replacement for endocarditis and pericardial patch repair of a subcoronary abscess cavity. The patch had partially dehisced, generating a supra-annular/subcoronary pseudoaneurysm. The CT demonstrates a largely thrombosed pseudoaneurysm of the aortic root at the right sinus of Valsalva (arrows). The right coronary artery (RCA) is draped over the pseudoaneurysm (right lower panel).

CHAPTER 4.1.7, REFERENCES 172, 173

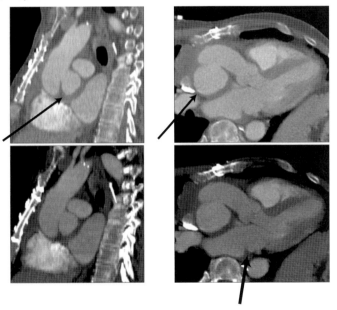

Figure 257   Postoperative pseudoaneurysm (4)

Format: MPR, MIP

This figure shows images of a patient with a history of orthotopic heart transplantation. There is a large pseudoaneurysm of the ascending aorta at the anastomosis site, with a maximum size of 6.2 cm (thin arrows). The typical anastomosis site of the native and transplanted left atrium is seen (thick arrow).

CHAPTER 4.1.7, REFERENCES 172, 173

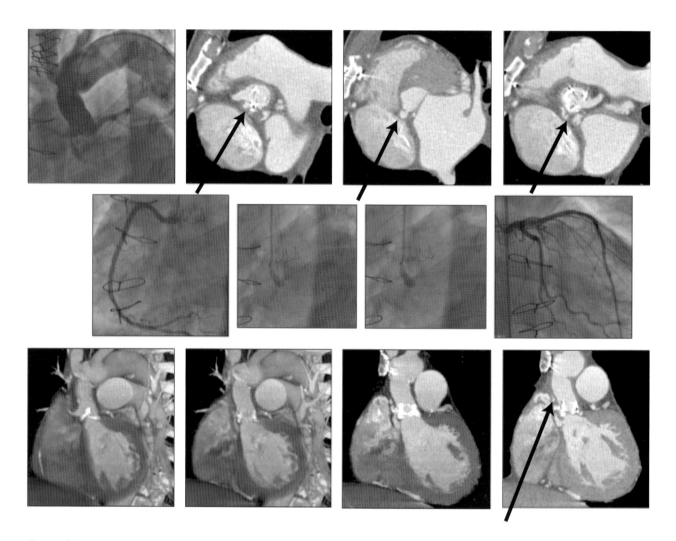

Figure 258   Paravalvular leak with small fistula of the aortic valve

Format: angiogram, MPR, VRI

This figure shows images of a patient with a remote history of aortic valve replacement using a composite graft (aortic valve and graft of the ascending aorta) with reimplantation of the coronary arteries.

During cardiac catheterization, a paravalvular tract was observed (left upper panel, and middle panels).

The CT images show evidence of aortic valve replacement with a valved conduit (arrow, lower right panel). There is paravalvular leakage beginning adjacent to the origin of the right coronary artery and draining into the left ventricular outflow tract as a fistula (arrows, upper panels). There is mild dilatation of the left ventricle.

CHAPTER 4.1.7, REFERENCES 172, 173

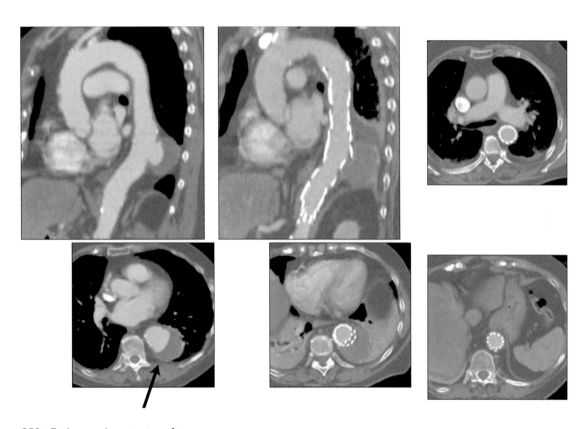

Figure 259   Endovascular stent graft

Format: MPR

CT imaging of the aorta is an integral part of endovascular stent graft therapy of aortic aneurysms.

This figure shows images of a patient with a focal pseudoaneurysm of the descending thoracic aorta (left upper and lower panels, arrow). The aorta at the level of the pseudoaneurysm measures 6.9 × 5.0 cm. The patient was treated with an endovascular stent graft (middle and right panels). The endovascular stent graft series extends from the proximal descending thoracic aorta to the level just above the celiac artery. The stent successfully excludes the aneurysm sac of the retrocardiac descending thoracic aorta. There is no peri-stent flow.

CHAPTER 4.1.7, REFERENCES 172, 173, 182–185

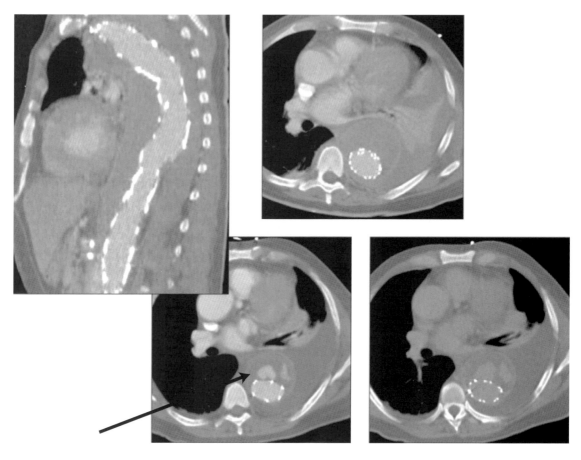

Figure 260 Persistent flow

Format: MPR

This figure shows images of a patient who was treated with a repeat endovascular stent procedure for persistent peri-stent flow. The lower images show the areas of persistent flow after the initial procedure: left lower, arterial phase (arrow); right lower, venous phase. After repeat stenting no flow is seen in the same area (upper panels).

CHAPTER 4.1.7, REFERENCES 172, 173, 182–185

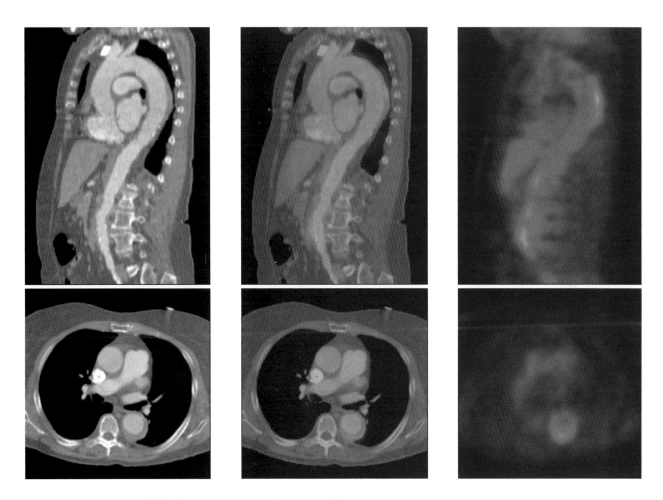

Figure 261   Aortitis PET/CT (see also color section on p. 17)

Format: MPR, scintigraphy

The morphologic changes associated with aortitis in the context of connective-tissue diseases can be assessed with CT. Typical findings are wall thickening and extensive calcification in later stages. The potential role of PET/CT scanners for the assessment of disease activity is currently being evaluated.

This figure shows MDCT and PET images of a patient with aortitis. The CT demonstrates smooth wall thickening of the aorta compatible with aortitis. There is prominent wall thickening in the mid-lower descending thoracic aorta, with a maximum thickness of 1.2 cm. There is also prominent wall thickening of the aorta at the renal artery level, which is indistinguishable from a large amount of para-aortic soft tissue.

The metabolic PET demonstrates regions of moderately intense fluorodeoxyglucose (FDG) uptake associated with the descending thoracic aorta and segments of the abdominal aorta. These findings are consistent with hypermetabolic inflammatory changes involving the aorta.

CHAPTER 4.1.7, REFERENCES 172, 173

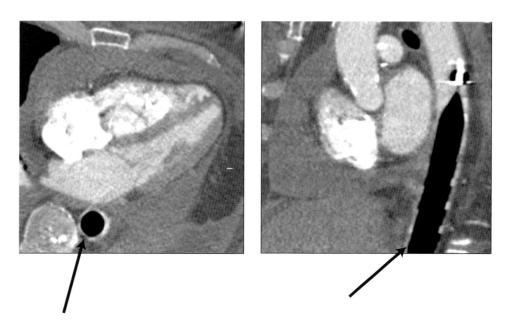

Figure 262   Intra-aortic balloon pump

Format: MPR

This figure shows images of a patient with a large pericardial effusion. In the descending aorta an intra-aortic balloon pump is seen (arrows). In the late diastolic images, the inflated balloon is seen in cross-sectional (left panel) and longitudinal (right panel) images.

CHAPTER 4.1.7, REFERENCES 172, 173

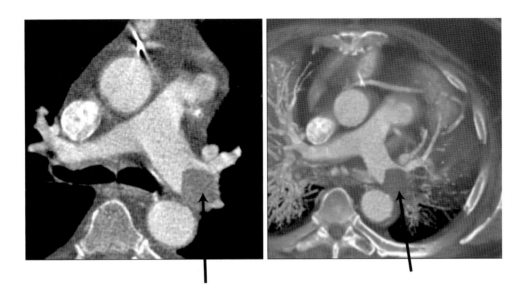

Figure 263 Pulmonary embolism

Format: MPR, VRI

Contrast-enhanced CT has a high sensitivity and specificity for diagnosis of proximal pulmonary embolus (main through-segmental arteries). This figure shows images of a large left central pulmonary embolus (arrows).

CHAPTER 4.1.8.1, REFERENCES 187–193

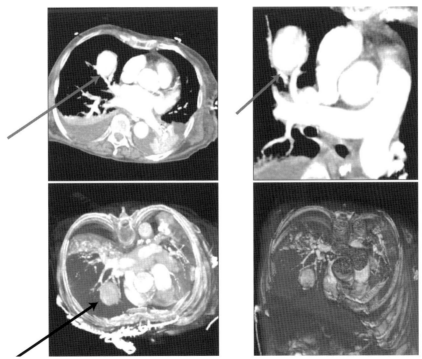

Figure 264 Pulmonary artery pseudoaneurysm (see also color scetion on p. 18)

Format: MPR, VRI

This figure shows images of a patient with a suspected pseudoaneurysm following the placement of a pulmonary artery catheter.

There are moderate bilateral pleural effusions with consolidation and atelectasis of the lower lobes. There is a pseudoaneurysm arising from the right middle lobe pulmonary artery, which measures approximately 4.0 × 3.3 cm (arrows).

CHAPTER 4.1.8.1, REFERENCES

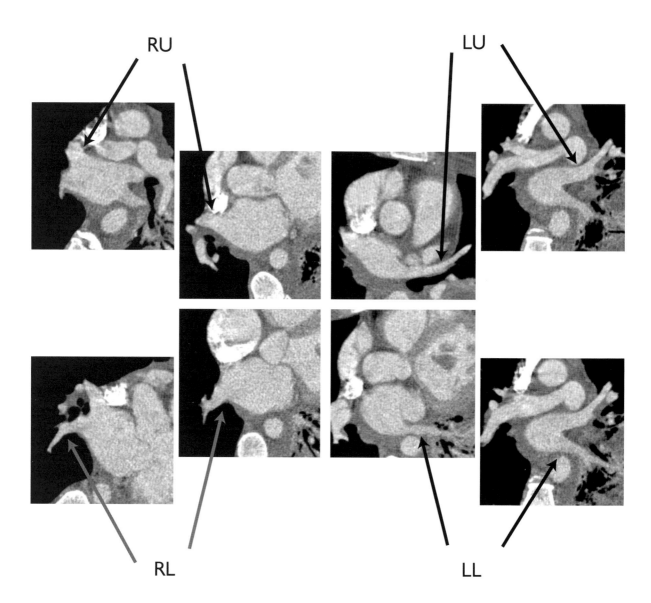

Figure 265   Normal pulmonary veins

Format: MPR

More recently, percutaneous ablation procedures at the pulmonary vein ostia have become a standard treatment for chronic atrial fibrillation in specialized clinical centers. Imaging of the pulmonary veins is now commonly performed before the procedure for guidance and after the procedure for diagnosis and surveillance of pulmonary vein stenosis.

This figure shows several images of the individual pulmonary veins entering the left atrium. The veins are normal. RU, right upper pulmonary vein ostium; LU, left upper pulmonary vein ostium; RL, right lower pulmonary vein ostium; LL, left lower pulmonary vein ostium.

CHAPTER 4.1.8.2, REFERENCES 194–197

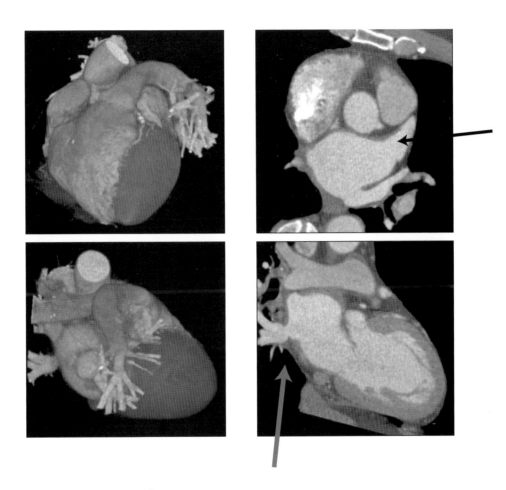

Figure 266   Pulmonary vein stenosis (1)

Format: MPR, VRI

Post-interventional imaging can assess complications, including wall thickening and luminal stenosis.

This figure shows images after pulmonary vein isolation (PVI). The left atrium and left atrial appendage show no evidence of thrombus (thin arrow). There is thickening of the vessel wall at the right inferior pulmonary vein ostium. This is associated with about 40% luminal stenosis (thick arrow).

CHAPTER 4.1.8.2, REFERENCES 194–197

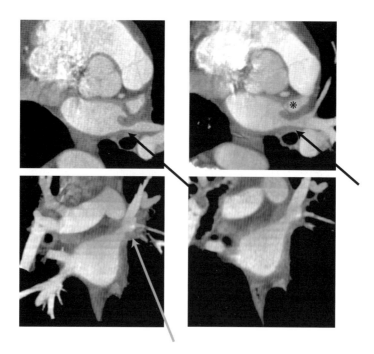

Figure 267   Pulmonary vein stenosis (2)

Format: MPR

More severe narrowing of the left superior vein ostium (arrows) is shown in this figure in a patient after pulmonary vein ablation. Note the location of the left atrial appendage (*) in relation to the proximal left superior vein ostium.

CHAPTER 4.1.8.2, REFERENCES 194–197

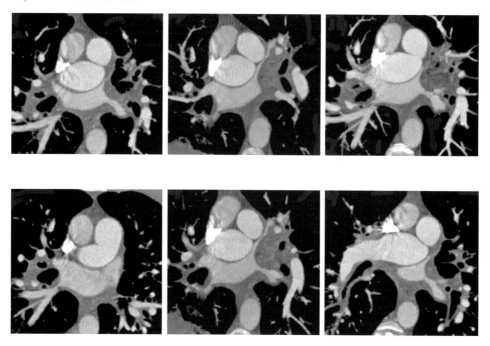

Figure 268   Pulmonary vein stenosis (3)

Format: MPR

An important advantage of CT is the ability to visualize inflammatory changes associated with the development of vein stenosis, including wall thickening at the vein ostia and mediastinal lymph node enlargement. This figure shows severe pulmonary vein stenosis of all four veins, with increased soft tissue in the mediastinum.

CHAPTER 4.1.8.2, REFERENCES 194–197

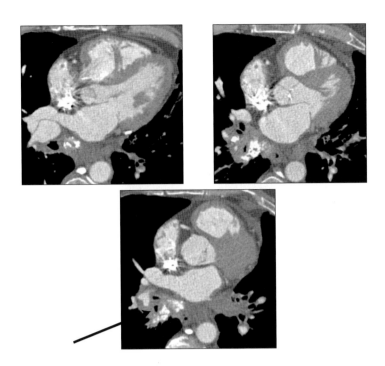

Figure 269   Fibrosing mediastinitis with pulmonary vein occlusion

Format: MPR

This figure shows images of a patient with fibrosing mediastinitis. There is partially calcified soft tissue in the mediastinum surrounding the left atrium (arrow). Only the right superior vein is patent. The other veins are occluded.

CHAPTER 4.1.8.2, REFERENCES 194–197

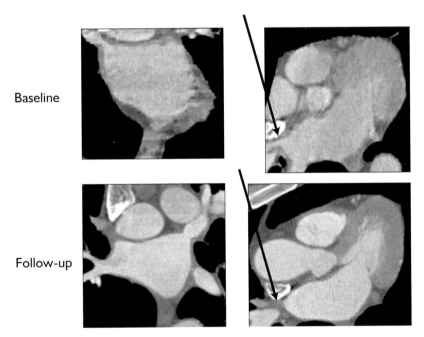

Baseline

Follow-up

Figure 270   Pulmonary vein occlusion (1)

Format: MPR

This figure shows images of two CT scans obtained 6 months apart. There is an increase in stenosis of the pulmonary vein ostia with total occlusion of the right superior vein ostium. The first scan, 1 month after ablation, showed 60% stenosis of the right superior vein ostium (arrow, upper panels). The follow-up scan 6 months later showed total occlusion of the right superior vein (arrow, lower panels).

CHAPTER 4.1.8.2, REFERENCES 194–197

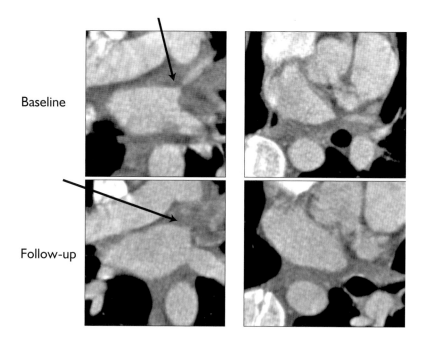

Figure 271   Pulmonary vein occlusion (2)

Format: MPR

In this figure, CT images 3 months (upper panels) and 6 months (lower panels) after vein ablation are shown. There is an increase in stenosis of the pulmonary vein ostia with total occlusion of the left superior vein ostium (arrows). However, it is important to consider that CT is limited in differentiating subtotal and total occlusion, which can be assessed with pulmonary angiography.

CHAPTER 4.1.8.2, REFERENCES 194–197

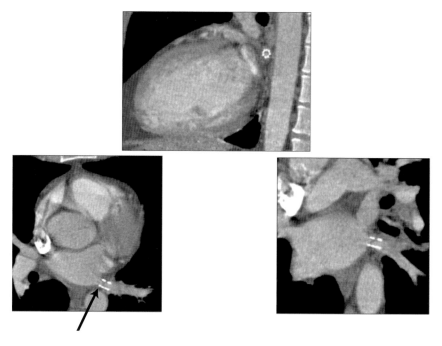

Figure 272   Pulmonary vein stent (1)

Format: MPR

Severe pulmonary vein stenosis is treated with angioplasty and stenting. Stent position and patency can be assessed with CT. This figure shows a patent stent in the left inferior pulmonary vein ostium (arrow).

CHAPTER 4.1.8.2, REFERENCES 194–197

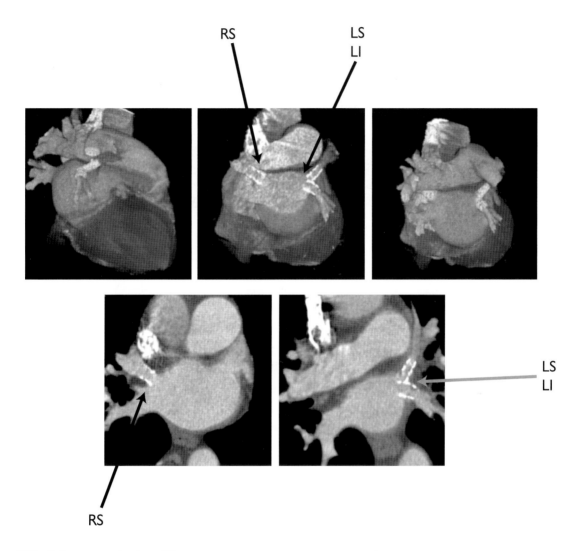

Figure 273   Pulmonary vein stent (2)

Format: MPR, VRI

Another example of stented pulmonary veins is shown in this figure. There are patent stents of the right superior (RS), left superior (LS) and left inferior (LI) veins. Both left-sided stents demonstrate small amounts of material lining the stent lumen. However, assessment of in-stent thrombosis or neointimal tissue inside the stents is limited with CT.

CHAPTER 4.1.8.2, REFERENCES 194–197

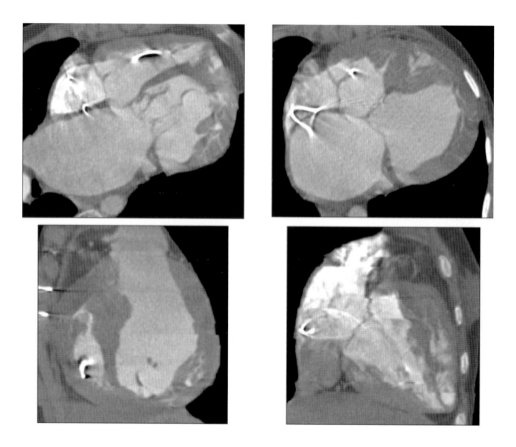

Figure 274   Congenitally corrected transposition of the great arteries (ccTGA) (1.1)

Format: MPR

MDCT is used in pediatric patients as a second-line imaging modality after echocardiography and MRI. However, if anatomic findings are unclear or confirmation is required, CT can frequently be performed with mild sedation because of the short acquisition time.

This figure shows images of a pediatric patient with congenitally corrected transposition of the great arteries (ccTGA) being evaluated for arterial switch procedure. Prior surgeries included pulmonary artery banding and closure of a ventricular septal defect.

There is thoracic and atrial situs solitus. There is normal systemic and pulmonary venous return. Atrioventricular discordance is seen with the right atrium communicating with the morphologic left ventricle, which gives rise to the pulmonary artery. The left atrium communicates with the morphologic right ventricle, which gives rise to the aorta on the left in a transposed fashion.

The left atrium and the morphologic right ventricle are enlarged. The septal component of the left-sided atrioventricular valve is apically displaced, compatible with epsteinoid changes. The morphologic left ventricle receives a pacing wire.

CHAPTER 4.2, REFERENCES 205, 206

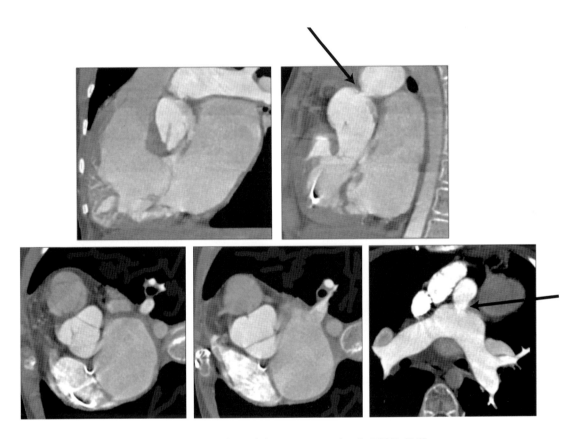

Figure 275 Congenitally corrected transposition of the great arteries (ccTGA) (1.2)

Format: MPR

The pulmonary artery has been banded beyond the sinuses (arrows). The coronary arteries originate from the base of the transposed aorta (lower middle panel) in an inverted fashion, with the artery to the morphologically left ventricle bifurcating into the LAD and LCX equivalents and the other artery following the left atrioventricular groove.

CHAPTER 4.2, REFERENCES 205, 206

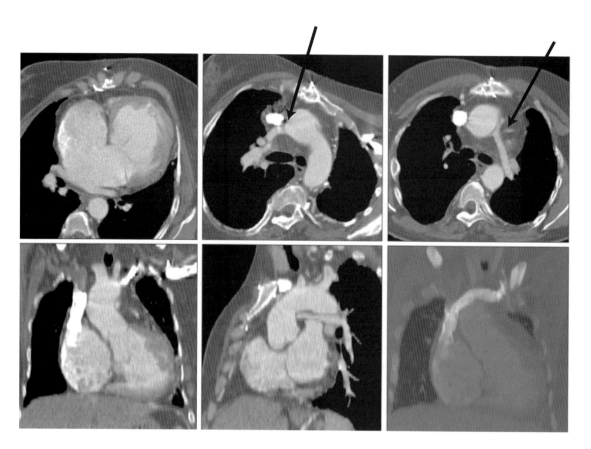

Figure 276   Tricuspid and pulmonary atresia

Format: MPR, MIP

This figure shows images of a patient with tricuspid atresia and pulmonary artery atresia, status post-central graft placement to the pulmonary arteries.

There are postsurgical changes in the thorax from prior open heart surgery. There is a single ventricle. There is a graft from the ascending aorta to the right pulmonary artery, which is patent (arrow, upper middle panel). An additional central graft to the left pulmonary artery is patent (arrow, upper right panel).

CHAPTER 4.2, REFERENCES 205, 206

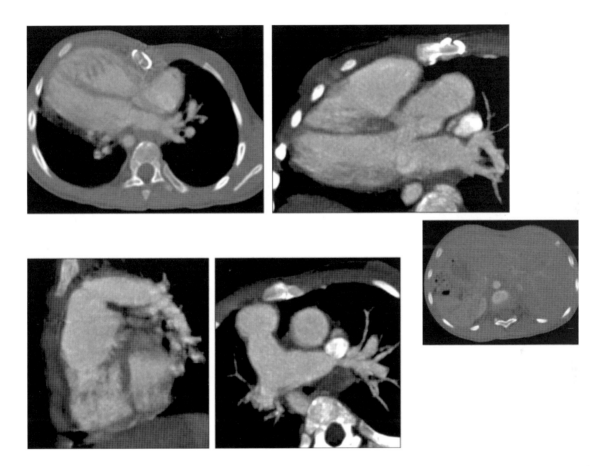

Figure 277   Situs inversus

Format: MIP

This figure shows images of a patient with situs inversus totalis. The heart is directed towards the right, and the liver is located in the left upper quadrant. There is additional evidence of surgical correction of the pulmonary outflow tract.

CHAPTER 4.2, REFERENCES 205, 206

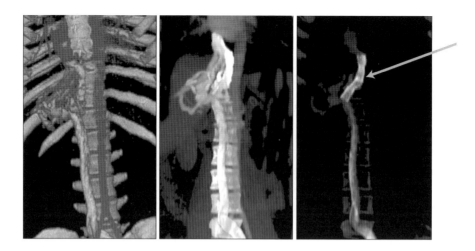

Figure 278   Stents in large collateral vessel of occluded inferior vena cava (see also color section on p. 18)

Format: VRI

This figure shows images of a 22-year-old patient with complex congenital heart disease, who presented with lower-extremity swelling. A work-up demonstrated that the inferior vena cava was completely obstructed and two overlapping stents were placed within large collateral vessels at the level of the obstructed inferior vena cava.

The current examination was performed for follow-up 2 months after stent placement. Contrast injection was performed from a foot vein. Two vascular stents are seen extending over a length of 8 cm at the level of vertebral bodies T9–T11 (arrow, right panel). At the level of the stents, just below the level of the hepatic veins, multiple collateral vessels are identified around the level of the IVC obstruction.

CHAPTER 4.2.9, REFERENCES 205–207

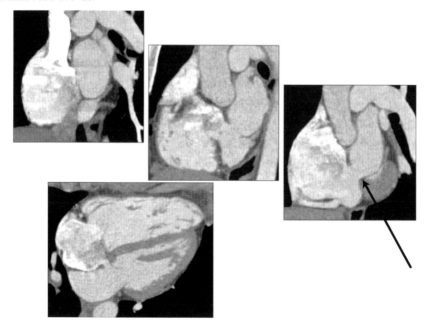

Figure 279   Coronary sinus atrial septal defect (ASD)

Format: MPR

Because of the thin, membranous structure of the central intra-atrial septum, anatomic assessment with imaging modalities is limited. Identification of atrial septal defects therefore relies on the assessment of flow with echocardiography and MRI. However, anatomic assessment with CT can define the relationship of the ASD to other anatomic structures, including the coronary sinus or the sinus venosus.

This figure shows images of a coronary sinus ASD. There is an unroofed coronary sinus, with a resulting ASD measuring 1.6 × 1 cm (arrow). There is mild right atrial and right ventricular enlargement.

CHAPTER 4.2.1, REFERENCES 205–207

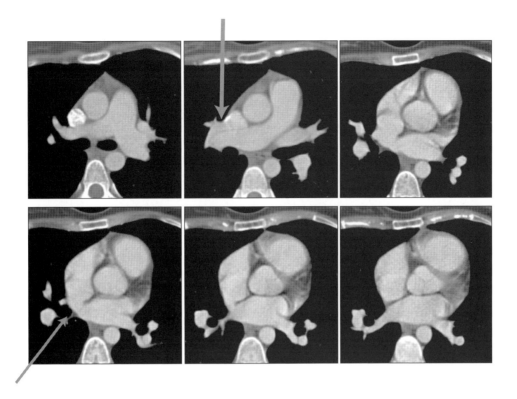

Figure 280   Sinus venosus atrial septal defect (ASD)

Format: MPR

This figure shows images of a sinus venosus-type atrial septal defect (thin arrow). The defect is located at the root of the intra-atrial septum. There is partial anomalous venous return involving the superior right pulmonary vein, which empties into the superior vena cava (thick arrow).

CHAPTER 4.2.1, REFERENCES 205–207

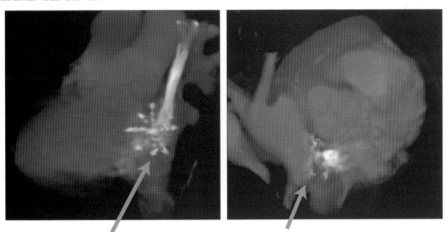

Figure 281   Percutaneous atrial septal defect (ASD) closure

Format: VRI

Surgical or percutaneous closure of atrial septal defects is considered depending on the clinical situation and anatomic characteristics. Recently, CT is increasingly being used for pre- and post-interventional imaging in the setting of percutaneous closure.

This figure shows post-interventional images after patent foramen ovale (PFO) closure with a #33 CardioSEAL® device. The cardiac structures are faded in this volume-rendered image. The high-density metal struts are clearly seen in relation to the surrounding structures (arrows).

CHAPTER 4.2.1, REFERENCES 205–207

227

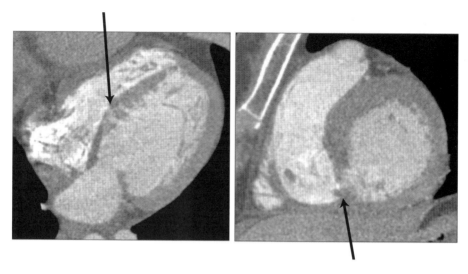

Figure 282   Ventricular septal defect (VSD)

Format: MPR

Ventricular septal defects are common in childhood but either close spontaneously or are closed surgically. They are therefore less commonly seen in adults. The different types of VSD (perimembranous VSD, muscular or apical VSD, inlet of atrioventricular canal VSD, supracristal of subaortic VSD) are related to the embryonic development of the interventricular septum. CT can identify the defect and describe the relationship to surrounding structures. Echocardiography, MRI and cardiac catheterization with evaluation of flow, pressure gradients and oxygen saturation is important for functional assessment.

This figure shows a small left ventricular septal defect (arrows).

CHAPTER 4.2.1, REFERENCES 205–207

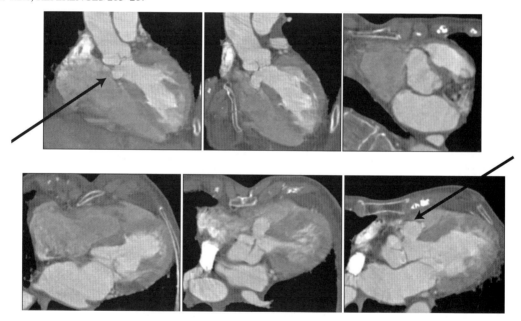

Figure 283   Aneurysm of interventricular septum: suspected spontaneous closure of VSD

Format: MPR

This figure shows images of a patient with suspected remote spontaneous closure of a ventricular septal defect (VSD). Below the right coronary sinus is a saccular outpouching of the left ventricular outflow tract, extending to the right atrioventricular groove (arrows). There is no communication to the right atrium or right ventricle. It measures 2 × 2 cm. The findings suggest an aneurysm of the membranous septum, probably secondary to remote closure of a VSD, with redundant tissue of the tricuspid valve.

CHAPTER 4.2.1, REFERENCES 205–207

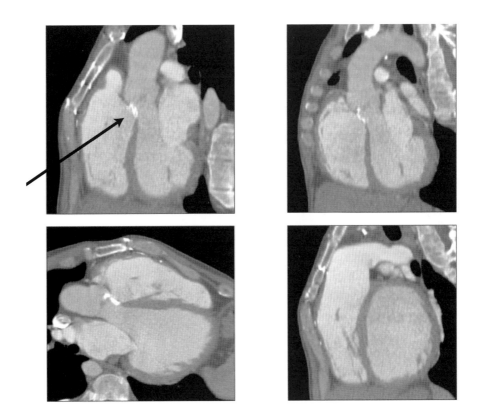

Figure 284   Repaired VSD in tetralogy of Fallot

Format: MPR

This figure shows images of a patient with repaired tetralogy of Fallot. There is dilatation of both ventricles. The patient has undergone reconstruction of the pulmonary outflow tract and closure of the ventricular septal defect with a patch (arrow).

CHAPTER 4.2.1, REFERENCES 205–207

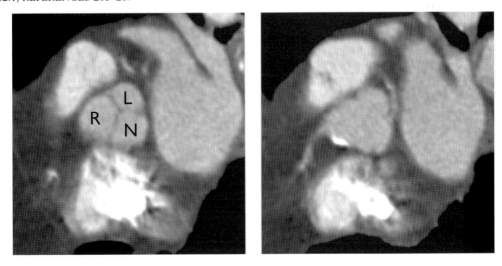

Figure 285   Anomalous coronary origin (1)

Format: MPR

An established application for CT angiography is the assessment of anomalous coronary arteries. Image reconstruction allows definition of the origin of anomalous arteries. The regular origins of the left main and right coronary arteries are the left and right coronary cusps, respectively. Variants without clinical significance are seen.

In this figure the left main coronary artery originates from the non-coronary instead of the left coronary cusp. N, non-coronary cusp; R, right coronary cusp; L, left coronary cusp.

CHAPTER 4.2.2, REFERENCES 208, 209

229

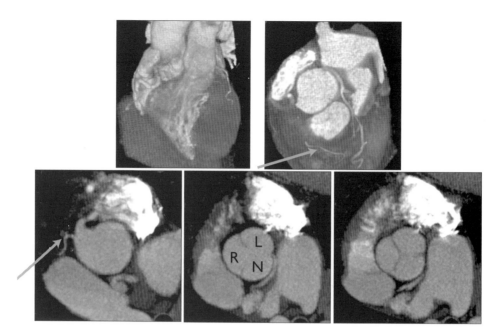

Figure 286   Anomalous coronary origin (2.1)

Format: MIP, VRI

Another example of an anomalous origin of the left main coronary (LM) from the non-coronary cusp – is shown in this figure. There is associated evidence of hypertrophic cardiomyopathy (see Figure 287).

The left main coronary artery arises from the non-coronary cusp adjacent to the left commissure and gives rise to the left circumflex (LCX) and the left anterior descending (LAD) coronary arteries. An additional left anterior descending coronary branch is supplied from the conus branch of the right coronary artery (arrows). No significant coronary atherosclerosis is noted. There is no evidence of myocardial bridge.

CHAPTER 4.2.2, REFERENCES 208, 209

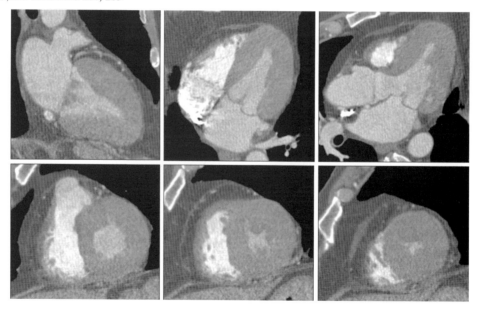

Figure 287   Anomalous coronary origin and hypertrophic cardiomyopathy (2.2)

Format: MIP

In addition to the anomalous coronary origin (see Figure 286), there is hypertrophic cardiomyopathy involving the mid- and apical left ventricular segments. The left ventricular outflow tract is not involved. There is thickening of the mitral valve leaflets with mitral valve prolapse.

CHAPTER 4.2.2, REFERENCES 208, 209

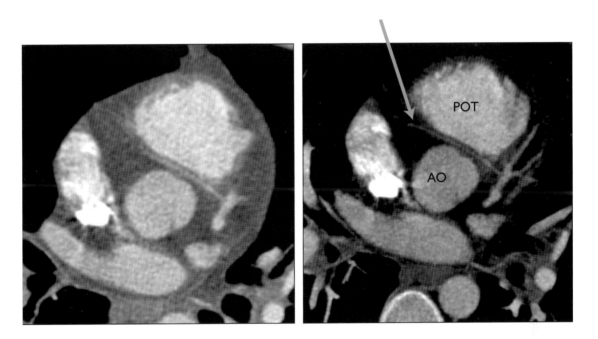

Figure 288   Anomalous origin of right coronary artery (RCA) of left main (LM) coronary artery (3)

Format: MPR, MIP

The origin of the right or left coronary system from the contralateral cusp or artery can have clinical significance. A course of the artery anterior to the aortic root, between the aortic root and pulmonary artery, is associated with possible systolic compression between the two structures.

In this figure, there is an anomalous origin of the right coronary artery from the left main artery. The RCA takes a course anterior to the aorta between the aorta (Ao) and pulmonary outflow tract (POT) (arrow). The RCA is a small, non-dominant vessel. There is no evidence of coronary atherosclerotic changes.

CHAPTER 4.2.2, REFERENCES 208, 209

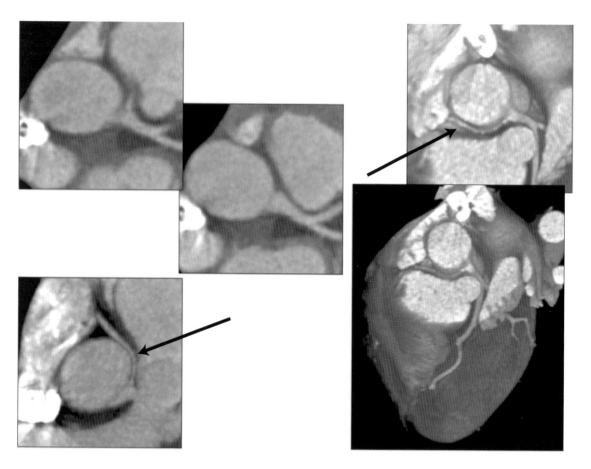

Figure 289   Anomalous RCA of LM (4)

Format: MPR, VRI

This figure shows images of a 15-year-old patient who was symptomatic with exertional chest pain.
The right coronary artery (RCA) originates from the left main coronary artery (LM). The RCA takes a course between the right ventricular outflow tract and the aorta (arrows) and continues in the right atrioventricular groove

CHAPTER 4.2.2, REFERENCES 208, 209

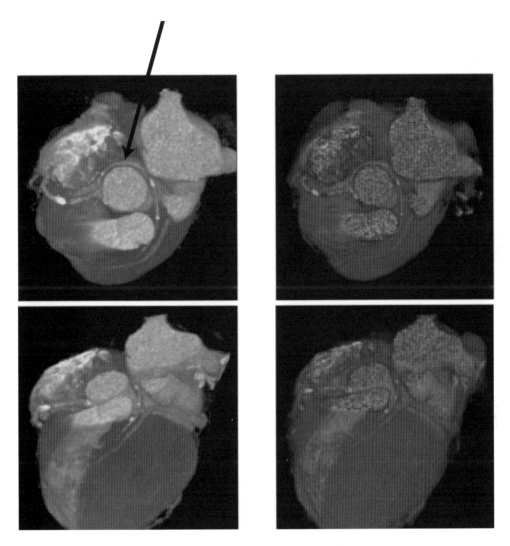

Figure 290 Anomalous coronary origin (5) (see also color section on p. 19)

Format: VRI

In this figure, the left and right coronary arteries originate with a common coronary ostium from the right coronary cusp. The left coronary artery then takes a course posterior to the aortic root, between the aortic root and the left atrium (arrow). Because the left atrium is a low-pressure system, this anomaly has a low risk of complications.

CHAPTER 4.2.2, REFERENCES 208, 209

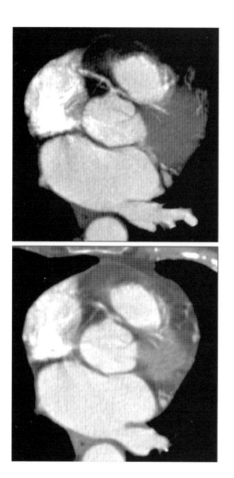

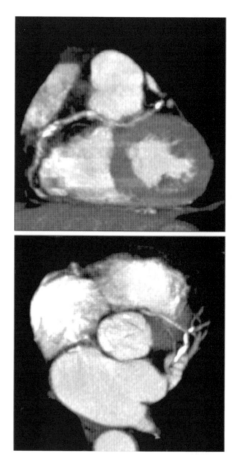

Figure 291   Anomalous coronary origin (6)

Format: MIP, MPR

As in the previous figure, the left coronary artery originates from a common origin with the right coronary artery of the right coronary cusp. However, the anomalous artery takes a course anterior to the aortic root, between the aorta and pulmonary artery. Because of the potential for systolic compression, the risk of complications is related to the course the artery takes between the aorta and pulmonary outflow tract/pulmonary artery. This is demonstrated in the following two figures.

It is also noteworthy that there is dense calcification of the right and left coronary arteries. The co-existence of a potentially significant coronary anomaly and potentially significant coronary artery disease complicates the further work-up of this patient with exertional chest pain.

CHAPTER 4.2.2, REFERENCES 208, 209

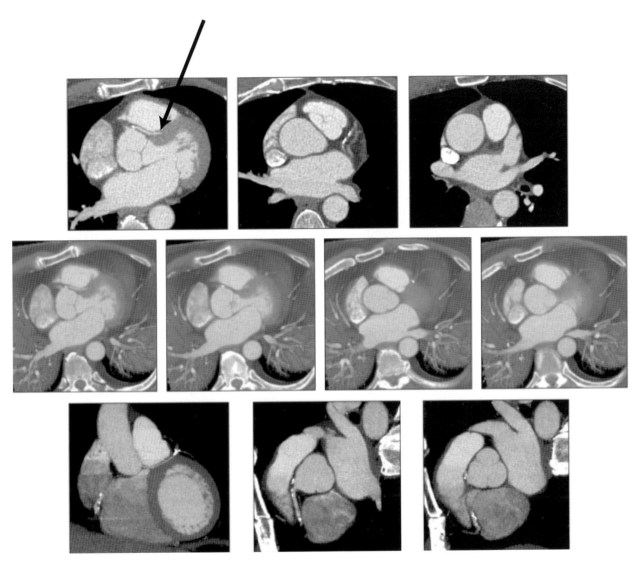

Figure 292   Anomalous coronary artery: intramyocardial course (7.1)

Format: MPR, MIP, VRI

As in the previous figure, the left coronary artery (LAD) originates from the right coronary cusp and takes a course anterior to the aortic root. However, the LAD crosses below the level of the pulmonary artery, between the aorta and pulmonary outflow tract. In fact, parts of the LAD cross in the high septal myocardium (intracristal course) (arrow). This anatomy is associated with a lower risk of systolic compression and clinical complications.

CHAPTER 4.2.2, REFERENCES 208, 209

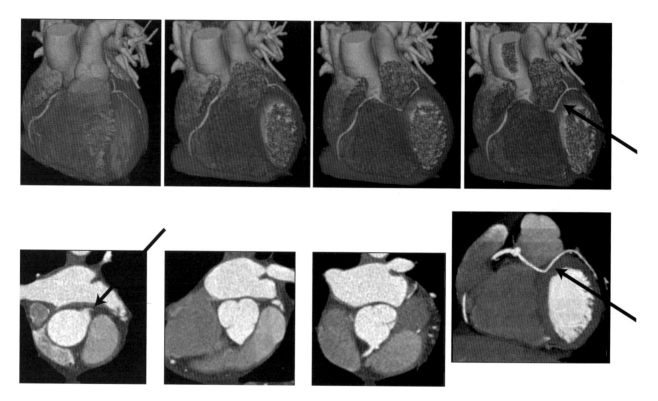

Figure 293   Anomalous coronary artery: intramyocardial course (7.2) (see also color section on p. 19)

Format: MPR, MIP, VRI

Another example of an intramyocardial course of the left main coronary artery is shown in this figure. There is an anomalous origin of the left main from the right coronary cusp, with a common ostium together with the right coronary artery. The left main then takes an inferior course below the level of the pulmonic valve in the interventricular septum between the left and right ventricular outflow tracts (thin arrows). The vessel resurfaces on the anterior aspect of the left ventricle and trifurcates into the LAD, a ramus intermedius and the left circumflex. There is a residual small branch originating from the left coronary cusp and termination in the proximal interventricular septum (thick arrow).

CHAPTER 4.2.2, REFERENCES 208, 209

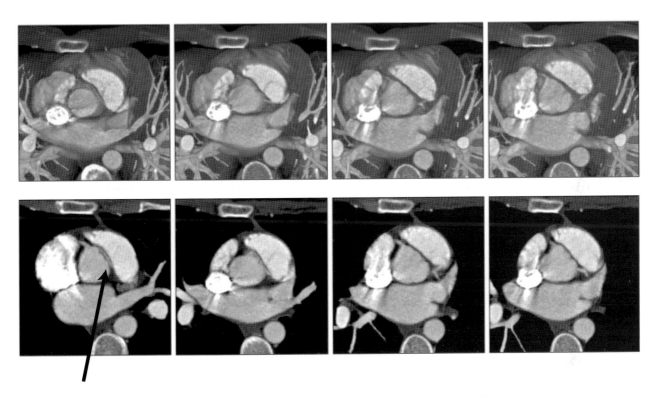

Figure 294   Anomalous coronary artery: course between aorta and pulmonary artery (8)

Format: MIP, VRI

As in the previous figure, the left coronary artery (LAD) originates from the right coronary cusp and takes a course anterior to the aortic root. However, the LAD crosses above the level of the pulmonary artery, between the aorta and pulmonary artery (arrow). This anatomy is associated with a higher risk of systolic compression and clinical complications.

CHAPTER 4.2.2, REFERENCES 208, 209

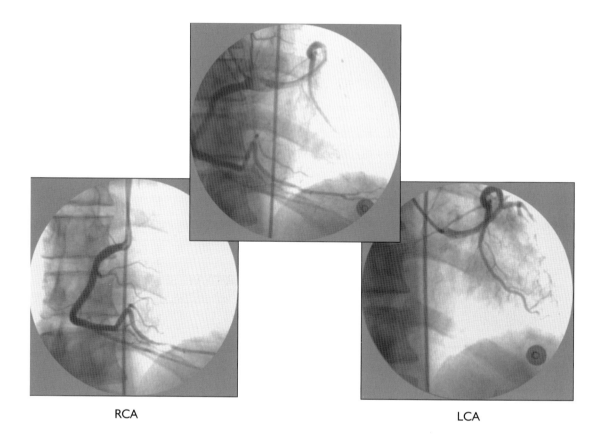

RCA   LCA

Figure 295   Anomalous coronary artery (9.1)

Format: angiogram

The complementary information of conventional angiography and CT imaging in the evaluation of patients with coronary anomalies is demonstrated in the next three figures. The angiogram shows the origin of the left anterior descending (LAD) and the right coronary artery (RCA) from a common ostium in the right coronary cusp.

CHAPTER 4.2.2, REFERENCES 208, 209

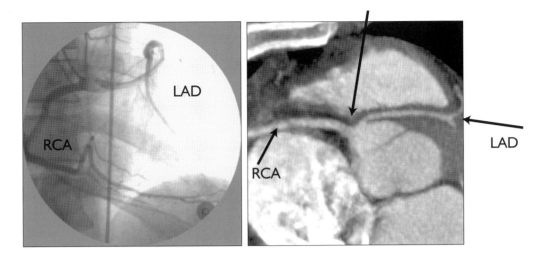

Figure 296 Anomalous coronary artery (9.2)

Format: MPR, angiogram

This figure compares angiographic and CT images. The CT demonstrates the origin of the left coronary system from the right coronary sinus of Valsalva. There is a common ostium (arrow) shared by the left coronary system and the right coronary artery (RCA). The anomalous left main coronary artery (LM) takes a course between the aortic root and the outflow tract of the right ventricle within the musculature of the crista of the upper interventricular septum.

CHAPTER 4.2.2, REFERENCES 208, 209

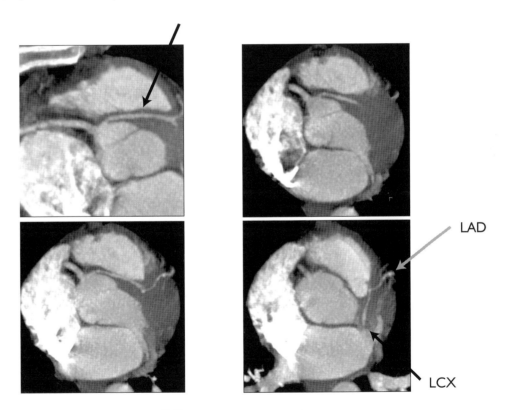

Figure 297 Anomalous coronary artery (9.3)

Format: MIP

Additional images show the origin and proximal course of the anomalous left coronary artery (arrow). In addition, the more distal course and bifurcation into the left anterior descending (LAD) and the left circumflex (LCX) coronary artery is shown.

CHAPTER 4.2.2, REFERENCES 208, 209

239

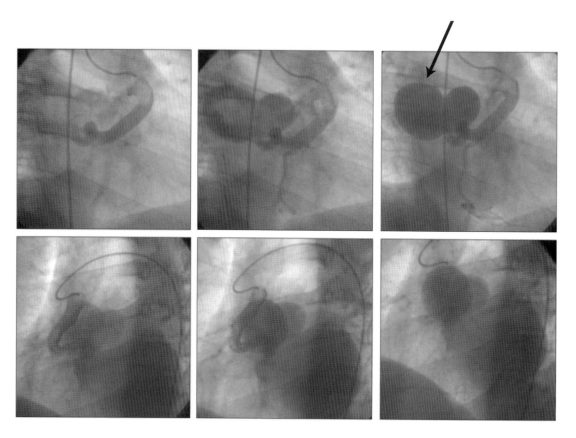

Figure 298   Coronary fistula (1.1)

Format: angiogram

CT can precisely describe the relationship of coronary anomalies to other cardiovascular structures. This information is complementary to conventional angiography. This becomes obvious in the assessment of a complex RCA fistula, as shown in the next three figures.

The conventional angiogram is shown in this figure. An enlarged fistula originates from the right coronary cusp and leads into a bell-shaped structure (arrow). There is filling of the left atrium (LA), probably secondary to communication between the fistula and the LA.

CHAPTER 4.2.2, REFERENCES 208, 209

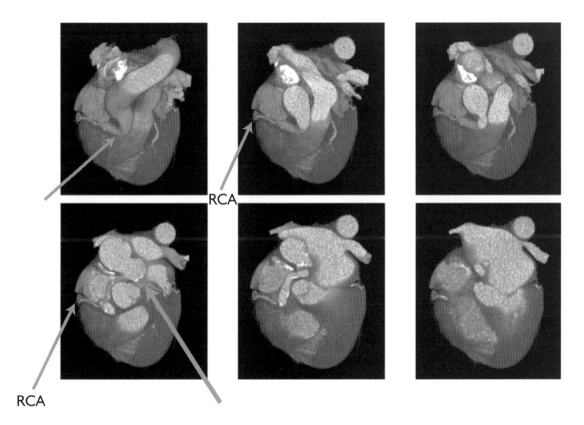

Figure 299   Coronary fistula (1.2)

Format: VRI

Corresponding CT images are shown in this figure. The origin of the fistula of the right coronary cusp is seen (thin arrow, left upper panel). The other panels show cut planes at different levels. The origin of the right coronary artery (RCA) and the connection of the fistula to the bell-shaped structure (thick arrow) are demonstrated.

CHAPTER 4.2.2, REFERENCES 208, 209

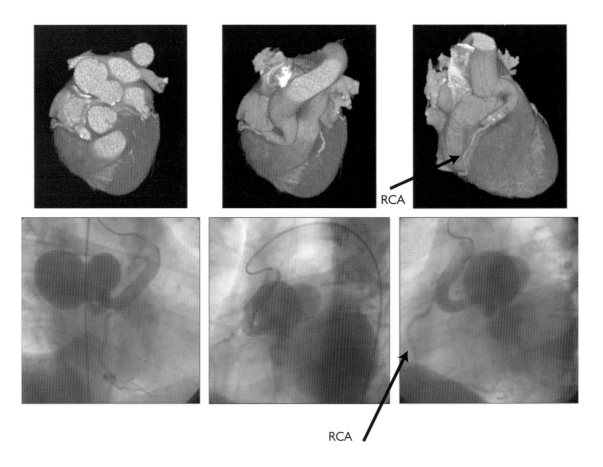

Figure 300   Coronary fistula (1.3)

Format: VRI, angiogram

Comparison between angiographic and CT images allows a better three-dimensional understanding of the RCA fistula.

CHAPTER 4.2.2, REFERENCES 208, 209

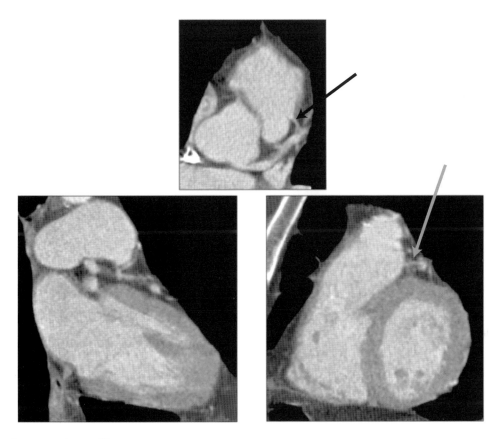

Figure 301   Coronary fistula (2)

Format: MPR

This figure shows small fistulas between the left anterior descending (LAD) and pulmonary arteries (arrows).

CHAPTER 4.2.2, REFERENCES 208, 209

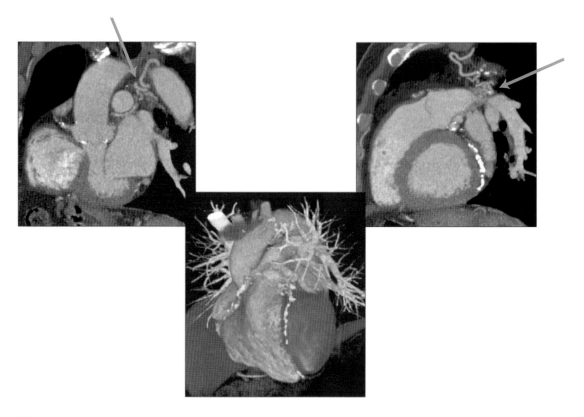

Figure 302 Coronary arteriovenous malformation (AVM) with connection to pulmonary artery (1.1)

Format: MIP, VIR

This figure shows an arteriovenous malformation (arrows) with contributions from the conus branch of the right coronary artery as well as the left main and left anterior descending coronary arteries. There appears to be an additional supply from a branch of the left internal mammary artery, although this is incompletely imaged. The malformation appears to drain into the pulmonary artery just above the pulmonary valve. There is coronary artery atherosclerosis.

CHAPTER 4.2.2, REFERENCES 208, 209

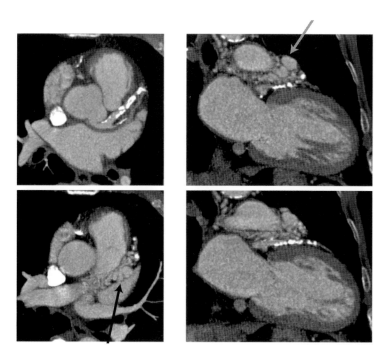

Figure 303   Coronary arteriovenous malformation (AVM) with connection to pulmonary artery (1.2)

Format: MIP

This figure demonstrates the vessel tangle located between the proximal left anterior descending coronary artery and pulmonary artery (arrows).

CHAPTER 4.2.2, REFERENCES 208, 209

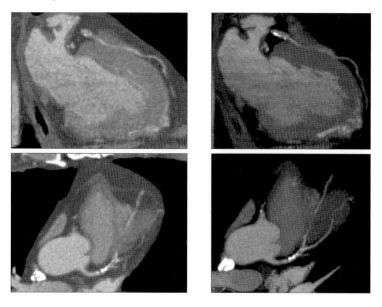

Figure 304   Myocardial bridge

Format: MPR, MIP

The large branches of the coronary arteries are located in the epicardial fat. However, individual segments occasionally have an intramyocardial location (myocardial bridge). MDCT permits the evaluation of these segments but cannot demonstrate the compression during systole, which is shown during conventional angiography.

An example is shown in this figure. The proximal LAD has a brief intramyocardial course consistent with a myocardial bridge (arrow). There are calcified atherosclerotic changes in the proximal LAD. Typically, the intramyocardial segment is spared.

CHAPTER 4.2.2, REFERENCES 208, 209

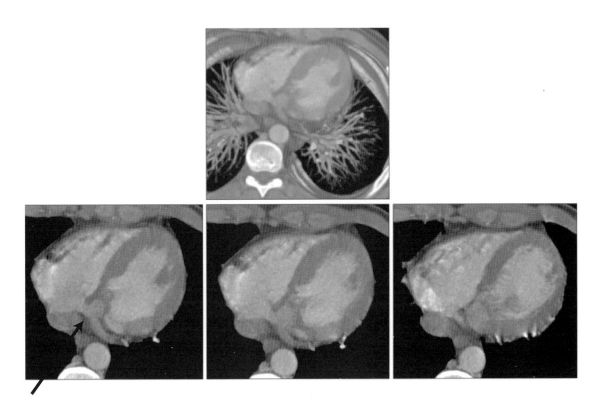

Figure 305　Sinus venosus aneurysm

Format: MPR, VRI

Abnormal coronary sinus anatomy, including coronary sinus aneurysms, can be visualized. The images in this figure show a coronary sinus with normal proximal dimensions. However, shortly after the ostium there is aneurysmal dilatation with a maximum dimension of 2.5 × 1.7 cm at the base of the interventricular septum (arrow).

CHAPTER 4.2.3, REFERENCES 210

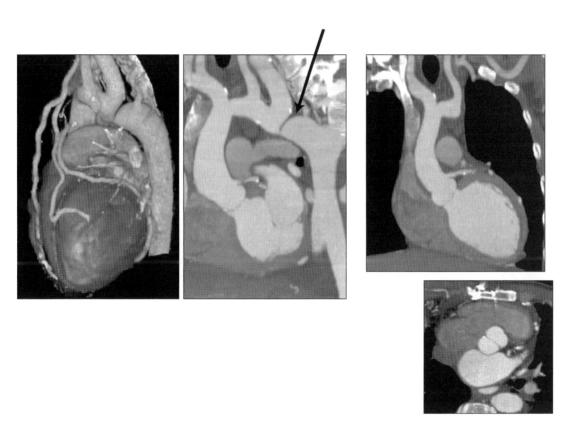

Figure 306   Coarctation of the aorta (1)

Format: MPR

In patients with coarctation of the aorta, CT can assess the anatomy and results after percutanous and surgical repair.
This figure shows images of a patient with a remote history of coronary bypass surgery. The CT scan demonstrates aortic
coarctation (arrow). There is hypoplasia of the arch with discrete juxtaductal narrowing of the isthmus. There are prominent
collaterals, including the internal mammary arteries.
In patients with aortic coarctation, the known association with a bicuspid aortic valve should be considered. In this patient,
fusion of the left and right coronary cusps consistent with a bicuspid valve was found (right lower panel).

CHAPTER 4.2.6, REFERENCES 211

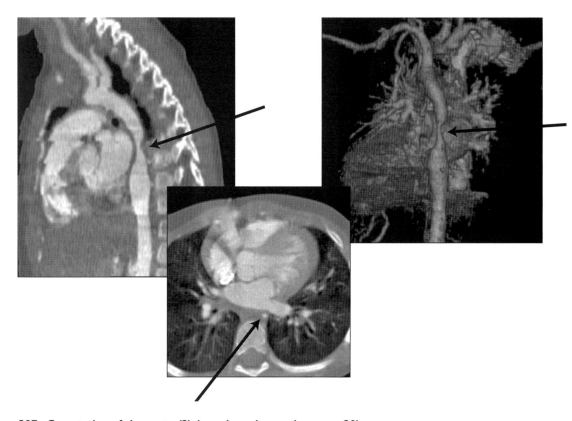

Figure 307   Coarctation of the aorta (2) (see also color section on p. 20)

Format: MPR, VRI

This figure shows images of a pediatric patient with aortic coarctation (arrows). Because of the young age of the patient, the scan was performed with the patient breathing and without ECG gating. Despite the resulting decrease in image quality, the images are diagnostic.

CHAPTER 4.2.6, REFERENCES 211

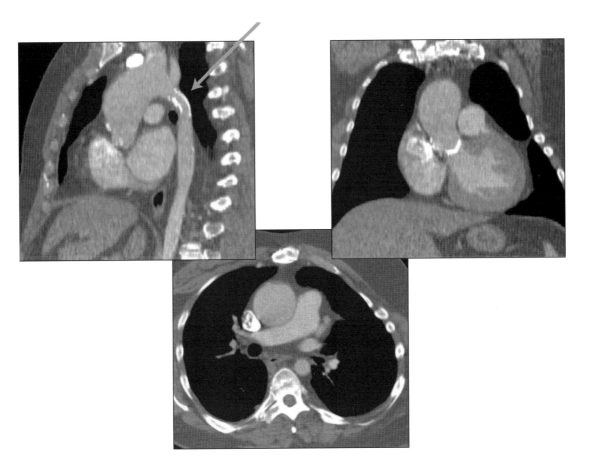

Figure 308   Coarctation of the aorta: stent (1)

Format: MIP

This figure shows images of a patient with a history of aortic coarctation and percutaneous repair with a stent.
There is replacement of the aortic valve with a low-profile mechanical prosthesis (right upper panel). There is fusiform
dilatation of the mid-ascending aorta with a maximum diameter of 5.3 cm. Prominence of the thoracic aorta continues into
the proximal arch, which has a diameter of 4.3 cm. Beyond the origin of the left subclavian artery, there is rapid tapering of
the isthmus to approximately 1.5 cm. An intact stent covering the area of the coarctation is seen (arrow).

CHAPTER 4.2.6, REFERENCES 211

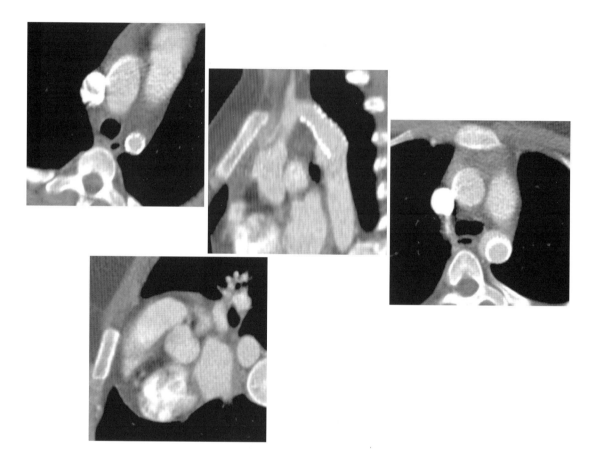

Figure 309   Coarctation of the aorta: stent (2)

Format: MPR

This figure shows images of a patient with a history of aortic coarctation, status post-remote surgical repair with a subclavian flap and subsequent stent placement for residual stenosis.

The aortic valve appears to be bicuspid (left lower panel), with fusion of the left and right coronary cusps. The aortic root has normal dimensions, measuring 2.7 cm. The sinotubular junction is maintained. There is a stent in the area of the proximal descending aorta. Minimal stent diameter in the proximal segment is 1.5 cm. At the distal end, the stent is not completely apposed to the aortic wall. In this segment, the native aorta measures 2.5 cm. The aorta then tapers to 1.8 cm in the mid-descending segment.

CHAPTER 4.2.6, REFERENCES 211

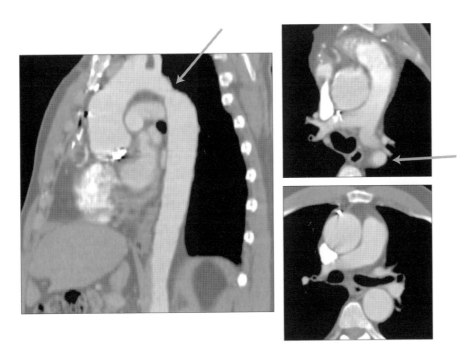

Figure 310   Coarctation of the aorta: surgical repair (1)

Format: MPR

This figure shows images of a patient with a history of surgical repair of aortic coarctation and aortic valve repair. There is evidence of end-to-end anastomosis of the aorta (arrows).

CHAPTER 4.2.6, REFERENCES 211

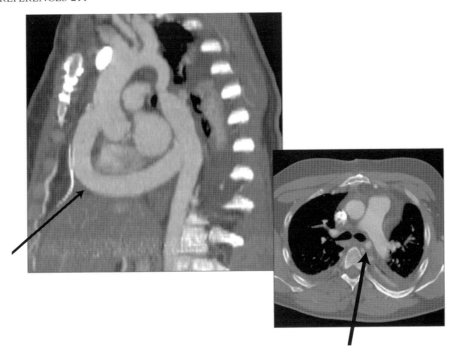

Figure 311   Coarctation of the aorta: surgical repair (2)

Format: MIP

This figure shows images of a patient with a history of surgical repair of aortic coarctation. There is a shunt graft extending from the ascending to the descending thoracic aorta (thin arrow). The narrowed area of the proximal descending aorta (thick arrow) is seen.

CHAPTER 4.2.6, REFERENCES 211

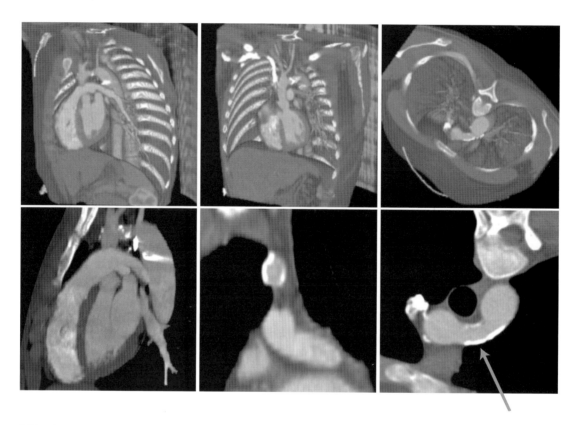

Figure 312 Grafted interrupted arch

Format: MPR, MIP, VRI

This figure shows images of a patient with a history of surgical repair for an interrupted aortic arch. There is an intact but calcified graft of the aortic arch, which measures 1.2 cm in diameter (arrow).

CHAPTER 4.2.6, REFERENCES 211

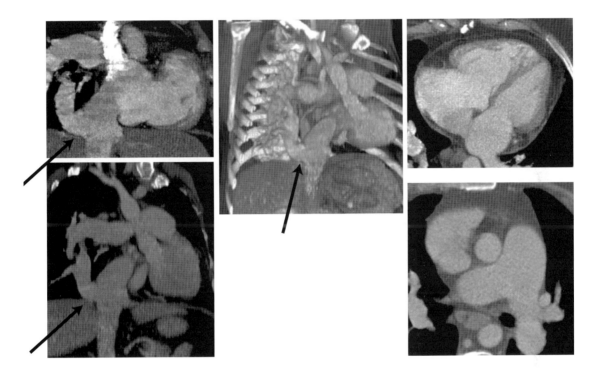

Figure 313 Partial anomalous return of pulmonary veins (scimitar syndrome)

Format: MPR, MIP, VRI

Partial anomalous return of the pulmonary veins is seen as an isolated finding or as part of other abnormalities.

There is anomalous pulmonary venous return of the right pulmonary veins to the inferior vena cava above the diaphragm (arrows). Together with hypoplasia of the right lung lobe, this finding is consistent with the scimitar syndrome. There is normal central venous return.

The cardiac chambers are notable for moderate-to-severe right atrial and right ventricular enlargement. There is severe dilatation of the central pulmonary artery, measuring 4.6 cm before the bifurcation (right lower panel).

CHAPTER 4.2.7, REFERENCES 205–207

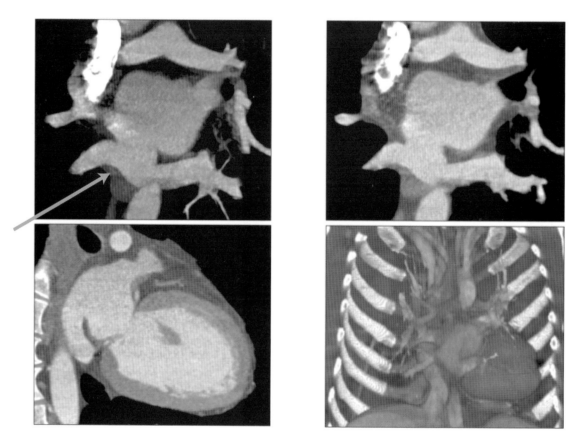

Figure 314   Corrected anomalous return of pulmonary veins

Format: MPR, MIP, VRI

This figure shows images of a patient with a history of surgical repair of total anomalous pulmonary venous return. The communication of the right and left pulmonary vein confluence with the anatomic left atrium is shown (arrow). The four major pulmonary veins are widely patent.

CHAPTER 4.2.7, REFERENCES 205–207

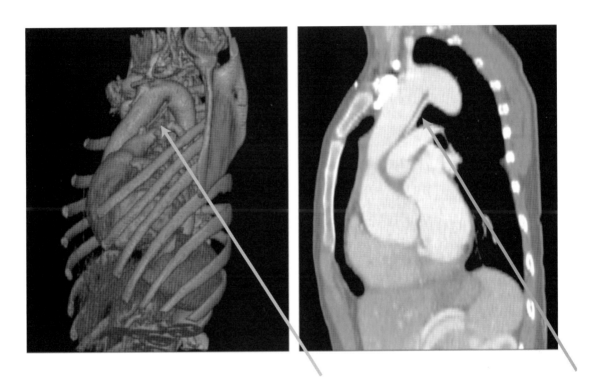

Figure 315 Patent ductus arteriosus (PDA) (see also color section on p. 20)

Format: MPR, VRI

The ductus arteriosus is a communication between the descending aorta (beyond left subclavian) and the main pulmonary artery (near bifurcation) and physiologically bypasses the pulmonary circulation in the fetus. A patent ductus can be found in asymptomatic adults, in particular if the size is small (arrows).

CHAPTER 4.2.8, REFERENCES 205–207

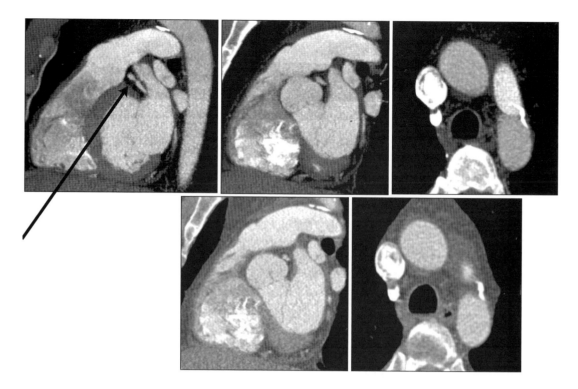

Figure 316   Spontaneous closure of ductus arteriosus: ligamentum arteriosum

Format: MPR, MIP

Physiologically, the ductus arteriosus closes after birth. The fibrotic remnant of the ductus arteriosus is called the ligamentum arteriosum. A calcified ligamentum arteriosum is shown in this figure (arrow).

CHAPTER 4.2.8, REFERENCES 205–207

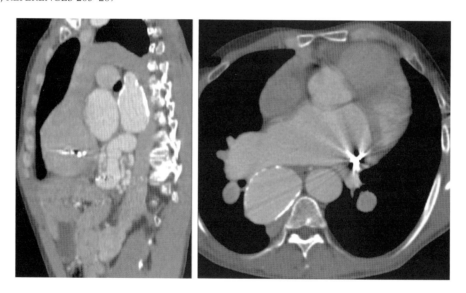

Figure 317   Complex arteriovenous malformation (1.1)

Format: MPR

This figure shows images of a large arteriovenous malformation with significant supply from a distal descending thoracic aortic branch and venous drainage into the left atrium. There is enlargement of both atria with a large arteriovenous malformation, that drains into the left atrium. There is a large supplying vessel in the distal descending thoracic aorta. Portions of this vascular malformation are calcified. There appear to be embolization coils in portions of the vascular malformation.

CHAPTER 4.2.8, REFERENCES 205–207

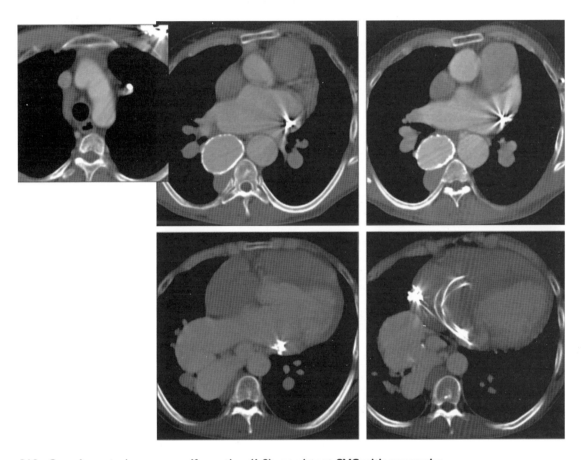

Figure 318   Complex arteriovenous malformation (1.2): persistent SVC with pacer wire

Format: MPR, MIP

In the same patient a persistent left superior vena cava connecting to the coronary sinus is demonstrated. Automatic implantable cardioverter defibrillator (AICD) or pacemaker wires pass through a persistent left superior vena cava and coronary sinus, and terminate in the right atrium and right ventricle.

CHAPTER 4.2.8, REFERENCES 205–207

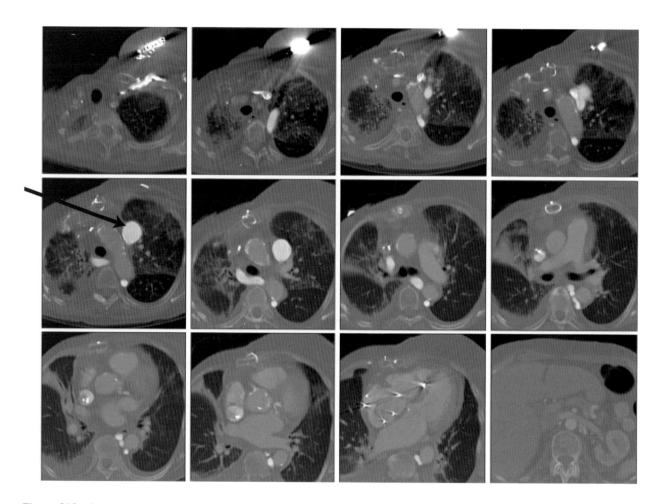

Figure 319   Aneurysm of persistent left superior vena cava (1.1)

Format: MPR

This figure shows images of a persistent left superior vena cava with aneurysmal dilatation adjacent to the aortic arch (arrow). The maximum diameter is 2.9 cm. The left superior vena cava drains into the hemiazygous system.

CHAPTER 4.2.9, REFERENCES 205–207

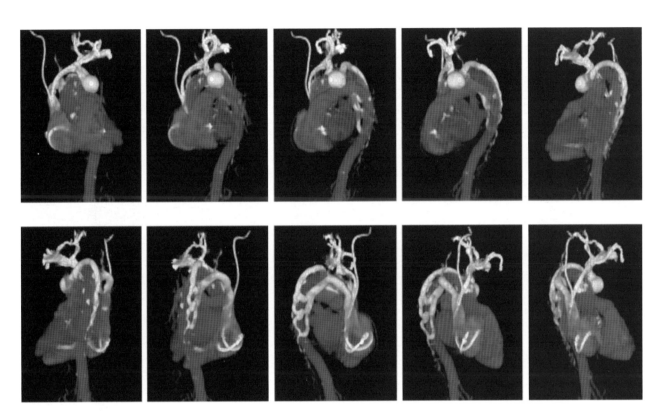

Figure 320 Aneurysm of persistent left superior vena cava (1.2)

Format: VRI

The venous anatomy and the aneurysm are also shown in this volume-rendered image.

CHAPTER 4.2.9, REFERENCES 205–207

5

Conclusion

Modern MDCT technology is used in a wide range of routine and emerging cardiovascular applications. Cardiovascular CT is complementary to other cardiovascular imaging modalities, including echocardiography (transthoracic, transesophageal, 3-D), a wide range of nuclear medicine techniques, angiographic techniques, magnetic resonance imaging (MRI), and ultrasound (US). The decision to utilize a particular modality should be based on the precise clinical question.

MDCT has already had a significant impact on cardiovascular imaging. Future developments will include advances in scanner technology and improved image analysis software, standardization of image acquisition and analysis. Eventually, guidelines for the use of cardiovascular MDCT, based on evidence from clinical imaging studies, will be formulated. We hope that this book reflects these developments.

6

Appendices

6.1   REPORT TEMPLATES

6.1.1   General requisition (MDCT scanner)

Hospital:
Patient name:
Identification #:
Clinical information:
Previous CT/MRI (attach report):
CONTRAST: YES/NO

CREATINE: DATE DRAWN:
ALLERGIES?

Gated spiral scan   3 mm slice thickness
                             1 mm slice thickness
Non-gated spiral scan   3 mm slice thickness
TIMING VESSEL
Ascending aorta   Descending aorta
Pulmonary artery
Left atrium   Left ventricle
Average of ascending aorta and pulmonary artery
CONCERN:
(1)   Thoracic aortic disease
(2)   Thoracic and abdominal disease
(3)   Coronary artery disease
(4)   Pulmonary vein abnormality
(5)   RV dysplasia
(6)   Pericardial disease
(7)   CAP stent protocol
(8)   Other
Contacts:

6.1.2   Assessment for aortic dissection

Hospital:
Patient name:
Identification #:
Ordering physician:
Test date:

Exam performed: CTA heart 3-D
Comparison: None
Clinical history: Patient presenting with chest pain suggesting aortic dissection.
Technique: Multidetector CT technology was employed. Spiral imaging with retrospective gating was performed following the intravenous administration of contrast material. Because of the patient's presumed cardiovascular disease history, a low-osmolar contrast agent was used.

For optimization of anatomic evaluation, advanced 3-D off-line post-processing was performed using multiplanar reconstructions, maximum-intensity projections and volume-rendered imaging.

Findings: The thoracic aorta has normal dimensions. There is no evidence of aneurysm, non-communicating dissecting intramural hematoma or communicating aortic dissection.

The cardiac chambers are normal and demonstrate no evidence of ischemic damage of the left ventricle. There is mild atherosclerotic plaque formation in the proximal LAD, but no evidence of significant occlusive coronary disease is seen.

The central pulmonary arteries are widely patent and show no evidence of pulmonary embolus. The lungs are clear. The mediastinum and pericardium are normal.

Impression: No evidence of significant thoracic aortic disease, including aortic dissection.

Principal investigator:

6.1.3 Postoperative report: recent open heart surgery

Hospital:
Patient name:
Identification #:
Ordering physician:
Test date:

Exam performed: CTA heart 3-D
Comparison: None
Clinical history: Postoperative evaluation, status post recent open heart surgery.
Technique: Multidetector CT technology was employed. Spiral imaging with retrospective gating was performed following the intravenous administration of contrast material. Because of the patient's cardiovascular disease history, a low-osmolar contrast agent was used.

For optimization of anatomic evaluation, advanced 3-D off-line post-processing was performed, using multiplanar reconstructions, maximum-intensity projections and volume-rendered reconstructions.
Findings: There are postsurgical changes in the thorax from recent open heart surgery. There are small bilateral pleural effusions and dependent atelectasis. The pericardium appears normal. There has been replacement of the aortic root with a Carpentier–Edwards prosthesis. Additionally, there is a supracoronary graft of the ascending aorta, which appears intact. There are the expected resolving blood products and a small amount of gas surrounding the grafted aorta.
Impression: No evidence of complications, status post recent open heart surgery.

Principal investigator:

6.1.4 Coronary bypass graft assessment

Hospital:
Patient name:
Identification #:
Ordering physician:
Test date:

Exam performed: CTA heart 3-D
Comparison: None

Clinical history: Patient with known coronary artery disease, status post coronary artery bypass grafting. There is concern for the status of the bypass grafts, prior to repeat bypass surgery.
Technique: Multidetector CT technology was employed. Spiral imaging with retrospective gating was performed following the intravenous administration of contrast material. Because of the patient's cardiovascular history, a low-osmolar contrast agent was used.

For optimization of anatomic evaluation, advanced 3-D off-line post-processing was performed, using multiplanar reconstructions, maximum-intensity projections and volume-rendered reconstructions.
Findings: An aorto-coronary saphenous vein graft (SVG) to the dominant right coronary artery is patent but has diffuse disease. A patent left internal mammary artery (LIMA) graft inserts into a diagonal branch of the LAD. Neither graft is in close relationship to the sternum. The native right internal mammary artery is intact without evidence of stenosis.

Diffuse, calcified atherosclerotic changes of the native coronary arteries are seen. There is no evidence of ischemic damage to the left ventricle.

The chest wall anatomy is notable for prior median sternotomy. The lungs are clear. The pericardium and mediastinum are normal.
Impression: Patent LIMA graft to LAD. Patent but diseased aorto-coronary SVG graft to the RCA.

Principal investigator:

6.1.5 Coronary artery assessment

Hospital:
Patient name:
Identification #:
Ordering physician:
Test date:

Exam performed: CTA heart 3-D
Comparison: None

Clinical history: Patient with positive risk factor profile for coronary artery disease, including family history and hypercholesterolemia. The patient is evaluated for a history of atypical chest pain. There is concern for coronary artery disease.
Technique: Multidetector CT technology was employed. Spiral imaging with retrospective gating was performed following the intravenous administration of contrast material. Because of the patient's

cardiovascular history, a low-osmolar contrast agent was used.

For optimization of anatomic evaluation, advanced 3-D off-line post-processing was performed, using multiplanar reconstructions, maximum-intensity projections, volume-rendered reconstructions and volume-rendered imaging.

Findings: Where visualized, the chest wall anatomy and lungs are normal. The pericardium and mediastinum are normal. The cardiac chambers are remarkable for concentric left ventricular hypertrophy. There is no evidence of myocardial ischemic damage. The visualized segments of the aorta are normal.

Coronary anatomy:

Left main coronary artery (LM): The left main trunk is a short vessel, which bifurcates into the LAD and circumflex. There is non-obstructive, non-calcified plaque accumulation in the distal segments of the left main trunk extending into the proximal LAD.

Left anterior descending coronary artery (LAD): The LAD is a normal-size vessel, which reaches the apex. It gives rise to a moderately sized diagonal branch. There is non-obstructive, calcified and non-calcified plaque accumulation at the ostium of the LAD and proximal segments of the LAD. At the origin of the first diagonal branch, there are complex atherosclerotic changes with dense calcification, which interferes with assessment of the degree of luminal narrowing in this region. Beyond this point, the mid-LAD has diffuse non-obstructive atherosclerotic changes. The first diagonal branch has diffuse, calcified atherosclerotic changes in its proximal section.

Left circumflex coronary artery (LCX): The left circumflex coronary artery is a non-dominant vessel that provides two lateral branches and a small-sized posterolateral branch. There is diffuse, non-obstructive calcified and non-calcified plaque accumulation in the proximal segments of the circumflex coronary artery. In the more distal segments, before the origin of the posterolateral branch, there are atherosclerotic changes with dense calcification. In that segment assessment of luminal dimensions/stenosis is limited.

Right coronary artery (RCA): The RCA is a dominant vessel. There is non-obstructive, non-calcified plaque accumulation at the ostium of the RCA. In the proximal segments, there is diffuse non-obstructive, calcified and non-calcified plaque accumulation. In the mid-RCA there are atherosclerotic changes with

dense calcifications. In that segment the assessment of luminal dimensions/stenosis is limited. The more distal segment has dense calcification.

Impression: Diffuse, atherosclerotic changes of all three coronary arteries as described above.

Focal, densely calcified atherosclerotic changes in the proximal-to-mid-LAD, distal circumflex and mid-RCA are noted, but the degree of calcification precludes precise assessment of the degree of luminal narrowing; functional assessment of the significance of these plaques is indicated using either stress echocardiography or nuclear imaging.

Principal investigator:

6.1.6 Pulmonary vein assessment

Hospital:
Patient name:
Identification #:
Ordering physician:
Test date:

Exam performed: CTA heart 3-D
Comparison: None
Clinical history: Patient with chronic atrial fibrillation, status post radiofrequency ablation/pulmonary vein isolation (RFA/PVI) at pulmonary vein ostia. There is concern for complications from the procedure, including pulmonary vein stenosis.

Technique: Multidetector CT technology was employed. Spiral imaging with retrospective gating was performed following the intravenous administration of contrast material. Because of the patient's history of arrhythmia, a low-osmolar contrast agent was used.

For optimization of anatomic evaluation, advanced 3-D off-line post-processing was performed, using multiplanar reconstructions, maximum-intensity projections and volume-rendered imaging.

Findings: Where visualized, the chest wall anatomy and lungs are normal. The pericardium and mediastinum are unremarkable. There is moderate left atrial dilatation. There are mild atherosclerotic changes of the coronary arteries.

The left atrium and left atrial appendage show no evidence of thrombus. There is mild wall thickening at the ostium of the left superior pulmonary vein. This is associated with a 35% stenosis at the ostium of the left superior vein. The luminal diameter is 1.2 cm. There is mild wall thickening at the ostium of the left inferior pulmonary vein, which is not associated with luminal stenosis. The right-sided veins are widely patent.

Impression: Mild wall thickening with associated mild luminal stenosis of the left superior pulmonary vein ostium. Mild wall thickening of the left inferior vein ostium without associated luminal stenosis. Patent right-sided pulmonary veins.

No evidence of left atrial thrombus.

Principal investigator:

6.1.7 Right ventricular dysplasia

Hospital
Patient name:
Identification #:
Ordering physician:
Test date:

Exam performed: CTA heart 3-D
Comparison: None
Clinical history: Patients with history of ventricular ectopy. There is concern for right ventricular dysplasia (ARVD).
Technique: Multidetector CT technology was employed. Spiral imaging with retrospective gating was performed following the intravenous administration of contrast material. Because of the patient's history of arrhythmia, a low-osmolar contrast agent was used.

For optimization of anatomic evaluation, advanced 3-D off-line post-processing was performed, using multiplanar reconstructions, maximum-intensity projections and volume-rendered reconstructions.

RV description: The right ventricular size is normal. There is no evidence of aneurysmal outpouching of the right ventricular wall. No definite evidence of fatty or fibrous replacement of the myocardium of the right ventricle is noted.

Miscellaneous: Where visualized, the chest wall anatomy and lung anatomy are normal. The mediastinum and pericardium appear to be normal. Left ventricular size, morphology and myocardial architecture are normal.

There is normal origin of the coronary arteries and there is no evidence of significant atherosclerotic coronary disease.

Impression: No imaging criteria of right ventricular dysplasia. Further evaluation with functional MRI can be performed if clinically indicated.

Principal investigator:

6.1.8 Assessment for congenital disease

Hospital:
Patient name:
Identification #:
Ordering physician:
Test date:

Exam performed: CTA heart 3-D
Comparison: None
Clinical history: Patient with history of tetralogy of Fallot; status post surgical repair. There is a need for assessment of cardiovascular anatomy in preparation for reoperation.
Technique: Multidetector CT technology was employed. Spiral imaging with retrospective gating was performed following the intravenous administration of contrast material. Because of the patient's presumed cardiovascular disease history, a low-osmolar contrast agent was used.

For optimization of anatomic evaluation, advanced 3-D off-line post-processing was performed, using multiplanar reconstructions, maximum-intensity projections and volume-rendered imaging.

Findings: The chest wall anatomy is notable for evidence of prior median sternotomy related to complete repair of the congenital condition. The lungs are clear. The pericardium and mediastinum are normal.

There is normal systemic and pulmonary venous return to the atria. Atrioventricular and ventriculo-arterial concordance is seen. In the left ventricular outflow tract there is a patch from remote repair of a ventricular septal defect. There is also evidence of surgical reconstruction of the right ventricular outflow tract with surgical widening by muscle resection. The right ventricle is moderately enlarged but shows no significant hypertrophy. There is also evidence of a remote right Blalock–Taussig shunt with interruption of the right subclavian artery and surgical anastomosis to the right pulmonary artery. The shunt is occluded. The right axillary artery appears to be reconstituted from collateralization and possible retrograde flow from the right vertebral artery.

The coronary arteries are notable for origin of the left main system from the posterior aspect of the left coronary sinus of Valsalva. Consequently, the left main coronary artery trunk passes between the posterior aspect of the aortic root and anterior to the left atrium before following an otherwise normal course.

The aortic arch is left-sided. The thoracic aorta is notable for only mild prominence of the aortic root and mid-ascending aorta, which both measure 3.7 cm but without significant annulo-aortic ectasia. The proximal arch tapers to 2.8 cm. The remainder of the thoracic aorta is normal.

The pulmonary arteries are notable for irregularity of the proximal to mid-left central pulmonary with moderate narrowing in its mid-portion.

Impression:

Evidence of remote Blalock–Taussig shunt (currently occluded) and complete repair with VSD patch and right ventricular outflow tract reconstruction.

Slight aortic root and mid-ascending aorta prominence but otherwise normal appearance of thoracic aorta.

Moderate narrowing of the left central pulmonary artery.

Principal investigator:

6.2 TEMPLATE FOR PHARMACOLOGICAL HEART RATE CONTROL

NOTE: The following pharmacological recommendations should be checked by a physician experienced in cardiovascular drug administration and adjusted to the specific clinical situation.

Utilization of intravenous beta-blockers (Lopressor®, metoprolol tartrate) during cardiac CT imaging
Effective date:

PURPOSE:

To decrease patient's heart rate and reduce RR interval variability for improved image quality from cardiac CT scans of coronary arteries. Goal to achieve is heart rate below 70 bpm.

CONTRAINDICATIONS:

Patients with congestive heart failure, asthma, bronchospastic disease, aortic stenosis, first-degree heart block, and patients currently taking beta-blockers, calcium-channel blockers (e.g. verapamil or diltiazem), or with a hypersensitivity to metoprolol. Use cautiously in diabetic patients, patients with hepatic insufficiency and those with peripheral vascular disease.

GUIDELINE/PROCEDURE:

(1) Place intravenous (IV) heplock (preferably #20 gauge) in patient's antecubital vein;

(2) Obtain two baseline blood pressures with heart rates;

(3) Inject 5 mg Lopressor IV slowly (over 3 min);

(4) Monitor blood pressure (BP) and heart rate (HR) frequently after injection;

(5) If target HR not obtained, may repeat dose of Lopressor 5 mg slowly IV × 2 (over 3 min) to a maximum total of 15 mg;

(6) Monitor patient's BP and HR every 5 mg frequently after injection;

(7) Physician may order nitroglycerin 1/150 tablet sublingual (SL) × 1 to be given immediately before CT scanning begins for coronary artery dilatation;

(8) Trained personnel and appropriate equipment for treatment of medication-symptomatic bradycardia must also be readily available.

6.3 TEMPLATE FOR PHARMACOLOGICAL VASODILATATION

NOTE: The following pharmacological recommendations should be checked by a physician experienced in cardiovascular drug administration and adjusted to the specific clinical situation.

Utilization of sublingual nitrates (nitroglycerin SL) during cardiac CT imaging
Effective date:

PURPOSE:

To increase the diameter of the coronary vessel in order to improve spatial resolution

CONTRAINDICATIONS:

Contraindicated in patients with hypersensitivity to organic nitrates, isosorbide, nitroglycerin or any component of the formulation; concurrent use with phosphodiesterase-5 (PDE-5) inhibitors (sildenafil, tadalafil, vardenafil); angle-closure glaucoma; head trauma or cerebral hemorrhage; or severe anemia.

GUIDELINE/PROCEDURE:

(1) Obtain baseline blood pressure (BP) and heart rate (HR);

(2) If the systolic blood pressure is 100 mmHg or greater administer 0.4 mg nitroglycerin SL immediately before the CT scan;

(3) Monitor BP and HR after administration.

6.4 TYPICAL SCAN PROTOCOLS FOR MDCT IMAGING OF VARIOUS CARDIAC INDICATIONS

Data are for a 16-slice scanner (Sensation 16; Siemens Medical Solutions, Erlangen, Germany).

	Coronary artery disease, myocardial disease, pericardial disease, valvular disease, cardiac masses, congenital heart disease	Coronary artery calcium screening	Thoracic aortic disease
Contrast enhancement	yes	no	yes
Acquisition mode	spiral	spiral	spiral
ECG referencing	retrospective gating	retrospective gating	retrospective gating
Cardiac phase	55% RR	55% RR	55% RR
Scan range	120 mm*	120 mm*	300 mm
Tube voltage	120 kV	120 kV	120 kV
Tube current	415 mA	137 mA	250 mA
Tube current–time product	620 mAs[†]	205 mAs*[†‡]	375 mAs[†]
Rotation time	375 ms	375 ms	375 ms
Temporal resolution	94–188 ms	94–188 ms	94–188 ms
Slices/rotation	16	16	16
Slice collimation	0.75 mm	1.5 mm	1.5 mm
Slice width	1 mm	3 mm	3 mm
Slice increment	0.5 mm	1.5 mm	3 mm
Table feed/rotation	3 mm	6 mm	6 mm
Matrix	512 × 512	512 × 512	512 × 512
Field of view	220 mm	260 mm	260 mm
Convolution kernel	B30f	B35f	B30f
Effective dose	14.2 mSv (F), 9.6 mSv (M)[§]	4.3 mSv (F), 2.9 mSv (M)[§]	15.1 mSv (F), 13.9 mSv (M)[§]

*Scan range may be increased for some indications with corresponding increase in radiation dose; [†]mA and mAs can be reduced on this scanner by approximately 50–65% using tube current modulation; [‡]mA and mAs are patient size-dependent and changed to maintain noise characteristics: value given is for average-size patient and may be increased or decreased for larger or smaller patients, respectively; [§]radiation exposure given in millisieverts and calculated using WinDose (Vers. 3.0; Scanditronix Wellhofer GmbH, Schwarzenbruck, Germany): value is reduced by approximately 33–50% using tube current modulation

References

1. Ambrose J, Hounsfield G. Computerized transverse axial tomography. Br J Radiol 1973; 46: 148–9.

2. Hounsfield GN. Computerized transverse axial scanning (tomography). Part I. Description of system. Br J Radiol 1973; 46: 1016.

3. Hounsfield GN. Computed medical imaging. Science 1980; 210: 22–8

4. Klingenbeck-Regn K, Flohr T, Ohnesorge B, et al. Strategies for cardiac CT imaging. Int J Cardiovasc Imag 2002; 18: 143–51.

5. Boyd DP, Lipton MJ. Cardiac computed tomography. Proc IEEE 1983; 71: 298–307.

6. Budoff MJ, Raggi P. Coronary artery disease progression assessed by electron-beam computed tomography. Am J Cardiol 2001; 88: 46E–50E.

7. Kalendar WA, Seissler W, Klotz E, Vock P. Spiral volumetric CT with single-breath-hold technique, continuous transport, and continuous scanner rotation. Radiology 1990; 176: 181–3.

8. Crawford CR, King KF. Computed tomography scanning with simultaneous patient translation. Med Phys 1990; 17: 967–82.

9. Woodhouse CE, Janowitz WR, Viamonte M. Coronary arteries: retrospective cardiac gating technique to reduce cardiac motion artifact at spiral CT. Radiology 1997; 204: 566–9.

10. Carr JJ, Crouse JR, Goff DC, et al. Evaluation of subsecond gated helical CT for quantification of coronary artery calcium and comparison with electron beam CT. Am J Roentgenol 2000; 174: 915–21.

11. Becker CR, Jakobs TF, Aydemir S, et al. Helical and single-slice conventional CT versus electron beam CT for the quantification of coronary artery calcification. Am J Roentgenol 2000; 174: 543–7.

12. Goldin JG, Yoon H, Greaser LE, et al. Spiral versus electron beam CT for coronary artery calcium scoring. Radiology 2001; 221: 213–21.

13. Budoff MJ, Mao S, Zalace CP, et al. Comparison of spiral and electron beam tomography in the evaluation of coronary calcification in asymptomatic persons. Int J Cardiol 2001; 77: 181–8.

14. Shemesh J, Apter S, Rozenman J, et al. Calcification of coronary arteries: detection and quantification with double-helix CT. Radiology 1995; 197: 779–83.

15. Broderick LS, Shemesh J, Wilensky RL, et al. Measurement of coronary artery calcium with double helical CT compared to coronary angiography: evaluation of CT scoring methods, interobserver variation, and reproducibility. Am J Radiol 1996; 167: 439–44.

16. Shemesh J, Apter S, Stroh CI, et al. Tracking coronary calcification by using dual-section spiral CT: a 3-year follow-up. Radiology 2000; 217: 461–5.

17. Klingenbeck-Regn K, Schaller S, Flohr T, et al. Subsecond multi-slice computed tomography: basics and applications. Eur J Radiol 1999; 31: 110–24.

18. Becker CR, Ohnesorge BM, Schroepf UJ, Reiser MF. Current development of cardiac imaging with multidetector-row CT. Eur J Radiol 2000; 36: 97–103.

19. Hu H, He HD, Foley WD, Fox SH. Four multidectector-row helical CT: image quality and volume coverage speed. Radiology 2000; 215: 55–62.

20. Fuchs TOJ, Kachelriess M, Kalendar WA. System performance of multislice spiral computed tomography. IEEE Eng Med Biol 2000; 19 (5): 63–70.

21. Flohr T, Stierstorfer K, Bruder H, et al. New technical developments in multislice CT, Part 1: Approaching

isotropic resolution with sub-millimeter 16-slice scanning. Rofo 2002; 174: 839–45.

22. Flohr T, Bruder H, Stierstorfer K, et al. New technical developments in multislice CT, Part 2: Sub-millimeter 16-slice scanning and increased gantry rotation speed for cardiac imaging. Rofo 2002; 174: 1022–7.

23. Flohr T, Kuttner A, Bruder H, et al. Performance evaluation of a multi-slice CT system with 16-slice detector and increased gantry rotation speed for isotropic submillimeter imaging of the heart. Herz 2003; 28: 7–19.

24. Fuchs T, Kachelriess M, Kalender WA. Technical advances in multi-slice spiral CT. Eur J Radiol 2000; 36: 69–73.

25. Nieman K, Cademartiri F, Lemos PA, et al. Reliable noninvasive coronary angiography with fast submillimeter multislice spiral computed tomo-graphy. Circulation 2002; 106: 2051–4.

26. Ning R, Chen B, Yu R, et al. Flat panel detector-based cone-beam volume CT angiography imaging: system evaluation. IEEE Trans Med Imag 2000; 19: 949–63.

27. Schoepf UJ, Becker CR, Ohnesorge BM, Yucel EK. CT of coronary artery disease. Radiology 2004; 232: 18–37.

28. Knollmann F, Pfoh A. Image in cardiovascular medicine: coronary artery imaging with flat-panel computed tomography. Circulation 2003; 107: 1209.

29. Vembar M, Garcia MJ, Heuscher DJ, et al. A dynamic approach to identifying desired physio-logical phases for cardiac imaging using multislice spiral CT. Med Phys 2003; 30: 1683–93.

30. Hong C, Becker CR, Huber A, et al. ECG-gated reconstructed multi-detector row CT coronary angiography: effect of varying trigger delay on image quality. Radiology 2001; 220: 712–17.

31. Kopp AF, Schroeder S, Kuettner A, et al. Coronary arteries: retrospectively ECG-gated multi-detector row CT angiography with selective optimization of the image reconstruction window. Radiology 2001; 221: 683–8.

32. Ohnesorge B, Flohr T, Becker C, et al. Cardiac imaging by means of electrocardiographically gated multisection spiral CT: initial experience. Radiology 2000; 217: 564–71.

33. Kachelriess M, Ulzheimer S, Kalendar WA. ECG-correlated image reconstruction from subsecond multi-slice spiral CT scans of the heart with subsecond multislice spiral CT. IEEE Trans Med Imag 2000; 27: 1881–902.

34. Flohr T, Ohnesorge B. Heart rate adaptive optimization of spatial and temporal resolution for electrocardiogram-gated multislice spiral CT of the heart. J Comput Assist Tomogr 2001; 25: 907–23.

35. Stierstorfer K, Flohr T, Bruder H. Segmented multiple plane reconstruction: a novel approximate reconstruction scheme for multi-slice spiral CT. Phys Med Biol 2002; 47: 2571–81.

36. Bruder H, Schaller S, Ohnesorge B, et al. High temporal resolution volume heart imaging with multirow computed tomography. J Electron Imag 1999; 3661: 420–32.

37. Boese JM, Bahner ML, Albers J, van Kaick G. Optimizing temporal resolution in CT with retrospective ECG gating. Radiologe 2000; 40: 123–9.

38. Halliburton SS, Stillman AE, Flohr T, et al. Do segmented reconstruction algorithms for cardiac multi-slice computed tomography improve image quality? Herz 2003; 28: 20–31.

39. Cohnen M, Poll L, Puettmann C, et al. Radiation exposure in multi-slice CT of the heart. Fortschr Roentgenstr 2001; 173: 295–9.

40. Morin RL, Gerber TC, McCollough CH. Radiation dose in computed tomography of the heart. Circulation 2003; 107: 917–22.

41. Hunold P, Vogt FM, Schmermund A, et al. Radiation exposure during cardiac CT: effective doses at multi-detector row CT and electron-beam CT. Radiology 2003; 226: 145–52.

42. Leung KC, Martin CJ. Effective doses for coronary angiography. Br J Radiol 1996; 69: 426–31.

43. Jakobs T, Becker CR, Ohnesorge B, et al. Multislice helical CT of the heart with retrospective ECG gating: reduction of radiation exposure by ECG-controlled tube current modulation. Eur Radiol 2002; 12: 1081–6.

44. Ho LM, Nelson RC, Thomas J, et al. Abdominal aortic aneurysms at multi-detector row helical CT: optimization with interactive determination of scanning delay and contrast medium dose. Radiology 2004; 232: 845–59.

45. Hopper KD, Mosher TJ, Kasales CJ, et al. Thoracic spiral CT: delivery of contrast material pushed with injectable saline solution in a power injector. Radiology 1997; 205: 269–71.

46. Haage P, Schmitz-Rode T, Hubner D, et al. Reduction of contrast material dose and artifacts by a saline flush using a double power injector in helical

CT of the thorax. Am J Roentgenol 2000; 174: 1049–53.

47. Irie T, Kajitani M, Yamaguchi M. Itai Y. Contrast-enhanced CT with saline flush technique using two automated injectors: how much contrast medium does it save? J Comput Assist Tomogr 2002; 26: 287–91.

48. Fleischmann D, Rubin GD, Bankier AA, Hittmair K. Improved uniformity of aortic enhancement with customized contrast medium injection protocols at CT angiography. Radiology 2000; 214: 363–71.

49. Bae KT, Tran HQ, Heiken JP. Multiphasic injection method for uniform prolonged vascular enhancement at CT angiography: pharmacokinetic analysis and experimental porcine model. Radiology 2000; 216: 872–80.

50. Gerber TC, Kuzo RS, Lane GE, et al. Image quality in a standardized algorithm for minimally invasive coronary angiography with multislice spiral computed tomography. J Comput Assist Tomogr 2003; 27: 62–9.

51. Schroeder S, Kopp AF, Kuettner A, et al. Influence of heart rate on vessels visibility in noninvasive coronary angiography using new multislice computed tomography. Experience in 94 patients. J Clin Imag 2002; 26: 106–11.

52. Blank M, Kalendar WA. Medical volume exploration: gaining insights virtually. Eur J Radiol 2000; 33: 161–9.

53. Mahnken AH, Wildberger JE, Sinha AM, et al. Value of 3D-volume rendering in the assessment of coronary arteries with retrospectively ECG-gated multislice spiral CT. Acta Radiol 2003; 44: 302–9.

54. Rubin GD, Beaulieu CF, Argiro V, et al. Perspective volume rendering of CT and MR images: applications for endoscopic imaging. Radiology 1996: 199: 321–30.

55. Sun Z, Gallagher E. Multislice CT virtual intra-vascular endoscopy for abdominal aortic aneurysm stent grafts. J Vasc Intervent Radiol 2004; 15: 961–70.

56. Saito K, Saito M, Komatu S, Ohtomo K. Real-time four-dimensional imaging of the heart with multi-detector row CT. Radiographics 2003; 23: E8–8.

57. Halliburton SS, Petersilka M, Schvartzman PR, et al. Evaluation of left ventricular dysfunction using multiphasic reconstructions of coronary multi-slice computed tomography data in patients with chronic ischemic heart disease: validation against cine magnetic resonance imaging. Int J Cardiovasc Imag 2003; 19: 73–83.

58. Choi HS, Choi BW, Choe KO, et al. Pitfalls, artifacts, and remedies in multi-detector row CT coronary angiography. Radiographics 2004; 24: 787–800.

59. Nieman K, Cademartiri F, Raaijmakers R, et al. Noninvasive angiographic evaluation of coronary stents with multi-slice spiral computed tomography. Herz 2003; 28: 136–42.

60. Goodenough DJ, Weaver KE, Costaridou H, et al. A new software correction approach to volume averaging artifacts in CT. Comput Radiol 1986; 10: 87–98.

61. Topol EJ. Textbook of Cardiovascular Medicine, 2nd edn. Philadelphia, PA: Lippincott Williams & Wilkins, 2002.

62. Braunwald E, Zipes DP. Heart Disease: A Textbook of Cardiovascular Medicine, 6th edn. Philadelphia, PA: WB Saunders, 2001.

63. Otto CM. Textbook of Clinical Echocardiography. Philadelphia, PA: WB Saunders, 2004.

64. Castillo E, Lima JAC, Bluemke DA. Regional myocardial function: advances in MR imaging and analysis. Radiographics 2003; 23 (Special issue): S127–40.

65. Boxt LM, Lipton MJ, Kwong RY, et al. Computed tomography for assessment of cardiac chambers, valves, myocardium and pericardium. Cardiol Clin 2003; 21: 561–85.

66. Kaminaga T, Naito H, Takamiya M, et al. Myocardial damage in patients with dilated cardiomyopathy: CT evaluation. J Comput Assist Tomogr 1994; 18: 393–7.

67. Juergens KU, Wessling J, Fallenberg EM, et al. Multislice cardiac spiral CT evaluation of atypical hypertrophic cardiomyopathy with a calcified left ventricular thrombus. J Comput Assist Tomogr 2000; 24: 688–90.

68. Vaitkus PT, Kussmaul WG. Constrictive pericarditis versus restrictive cardiomyopathy: a reappraisal and update of diagnostic criteria. Am Heart J 1991; 122: 1431–41.

69. Hulot JS, Jouven X, Empana JP, et al. Natural history and risk stratification of arrhythmogenic right ventricular dysplasia/cardiomyopathy. Circulation 2004; 110: 1879–84.

70. Marcus F, Towbin JA, Zareba W, et al.; ARVD/C Investigators. Arrhythmogenic right ventricular dysplasia/cardiomyopathy (ARVD/C): a multi-disciplinary study: design and protocol. Circulation 2003; 107: 2975–8.

71. Castillo E, Tandri H, Rodriguez ER, et al. Arrhythmogenic right ventricular dysplasia: ex vivo and in vivo fat detection with black-blood MR imaging. Radiology 2004; 232: 38–48.

72. Tandri H, Bomma C, Calkins H, Bluemke DA. Magnetic resonance and computed tomography imaging of arrhythmogenic right ventricular dysplasia. J Magn Reson Imag 2004; 19: 848–58.

73. Kayser HW, van der Wall EE, Sivananthan MU, et al. Diagnosis of arrhythmogenic right ventricular dysplasia: a review. Radiographics 2002; 22: 639–48.

74. Antman EM, Anbe DT, Armstrong PW, et al. American College of Cardiology; American Heart Association Task Force on Practice Guidelines; Canadian Cardiovascular Society. ACC/AHA guidelines for the management of patients with ST-elevation myocardial infarction: a report of the American College of Cardiology/American Heart Association Task Force on Practice Guidelines. Circulation 2004; 110: e82–292.

75. Naito H, Saito H, Takamiya M, et al. Quantitative assessment of myocardial enhancement with iodinated contrast medium in patient with ischemic heart disease by using ultrafast X-ray computed tomography. Invest Radiol 1992; 27: 436–42.

76. Gray WR Jr, Parkey RW, Buja LM, et al. Computed tomography: in vitro evaluation of myocardial infarction. Radiology 1977; 122: 511–13.

77. Hoffmann U, Millea R, Enzweiler C, et al. Acute myocardial infarction: contrast-enhanced multidetector row CT in a porcine model. Radiology 2004; 231: 697–701.

78. Feuchter GM, Friedrich GJ, Mallouhi A, zur Nedden D. Assessment of myocardial infarction with 16-channel multislice computed tomography. Int J Cardiovasc Imag 2004; 20: 416 (abstr 21).

79. Kim RJ, Fieno DS, Parrish TB, et al. Relationship of MRI delayed contrast enhancement to irreversible injury, infarct age, and contractile function. Circulation 1999; 100: 1992–2002.

80. Paul JF, Macé L, Caussin C, et al. Multirow detector computed tomography assessment of intraseptal dissection and ventricular pseudoaneurysm in postinfarction ventricular septal defect. Circulation 2001; 104: 497–8.

81. Lipton MJ, Bogaert J, Boxt LM, Reba RC. Imaging of ischemic heart disease. Eur Radiol 2002; 12: 1061–80.

82. Black IW, Stewart WJ. The role of echocardiography in the evaluation of cardiac source of embolism: left atrial spontaneous echo contrast. Echocardiography 1993; 10: 429–39.

83. Vincelj J, Sokol I, Jaksic O. Prevalence and clinical significance of left atrial spontaneous echo contrast detected by transesophageal echocardiography. Echocardiography 2002; 19: 319–24.

84. Sengupta PP, Mohan JC, Mehta V, et al. Comparison of echocardiographic features of noncompaction of the left ventricle in adults versus idiopathic dilated cardiomyopathy in adults. Am J Cardiol 2004; 94: 389–91.

85. Pignatelli RH, McMahon CJ, Dreyer WJ, et al. Clinical characterization of left ventricular noncompaction in children: a relatively common form of cardiomyopathy. Circulation 2003; 108: 2672–8.

86. Heyer CM, Kagel T, Lemburg SP, et al. Lipomatous hypertrophy of the interatrial septum: a prospective study of incidence, imaging findings, and clinical symptoms. Chest 2003; 124: 2068–73.

87. Meaney JF, Kazerooni EA, Jamadar DA, Korobkin M. CT appearance of lipomatous hypertrophy of the interatrial septum. Am J Roentgenol 1997; 168: 1081–4.

88. Friedrich MG, Strohm O, Schulz-Menger J, et al. Contrast media-enhanced magnetic resonance imaging visualizes myocardial changes in the course of viral myocarditis. Circulation 1998; 97: 1802–9.

89. De Feyter PJ, Nieman K. Noninvasive multi-slice computed tomography coronary angiography – an emerging clinical modality. J Am Coll Cardiol 2003; 44: 1238–40.

90. Schoenhagen P, Halliburton SS, Stillman AE, et al. Noninvasive imaging of coronary arteries: current and future role of multi-detector row CT. Radiology 2004; 232: 7–17.

91. Pannu HK, Flohr TG, Corl FM, Fishman EK. Current concepts in multi-detector row CT evaluation of the coronary arteries: principles, techniques, and anatomy. Radiographics 2003; 23 (Special issue): S111–25.

92. White RD, Setser RM. Integrated approach to evaluating coronary artery disease and ischemic heart disease. Am J Cardiol 2002; 90: 49L–55L.

93. Libby P. Current concepts of the pathogenesis of the acute coronary syndromes. Circulation 2001; 104: 365–72.

94. Topol EJ, Nissen SE. Our preoccupation with coronary luminology. Circulation 1995; 92: 2333–42.

95. Schoenhagen P, White RD, Nissen SE, Tuzcu EM. Coronary imaging: angiography shows the stenosis, but IVUS, CT, and MRI show the plaque. Cleve Clin J Med 2003; 70: 713–19.

96. Falk E, Shah PK, Fuster V. Coronary plaque disruption. Circulation 1995; 92: 657–71.

97. Fayad ZA, Fuster V. Clinical imaging of the high-risk or vulnerable atherosclerotic plaque. Circ Res 2001; 89: 305–16.

98. Schmermund A, Erbel R. Unstable coronary plaque and its relation to coronary calcium. Circulation 2001; 104: 1682–7.

99. Schoenhagen P, Tuzcu EM. Coronary artery calcification and end-stage renal disease: vascular biology and clinical implications. Cleve Clin J Med 2002; 69 (Suppl 3): S12–20.

100. Agatston AS, Janowitz WR, Hildner FJ, et al. Quantification of coronary artery calcium using ultrafast computed tomography. J Am Coll Cardiol 1990; 15: 827–32.

101. Shemesh J, Apter S, Rozenman J, et al. Calcification of coronary arteries. Radiology 1995; 197: 779–83.

102. Hoff JA, Chomka EV, Kranik AJ, et al. Age and gender distributions of coronary artery calcium detected by electron-beam tomography in 35 246 adults. Am J Cardiol 2001; 87: 1335–9.

103. Schmermund A, Erbel R, Silber S. Age and gender distribution of coonary artery calcium measured by four-slice computed tomography in 2030 persons with no symptoms of coronary artery disease. Am J Cardiol 2002; 90: 168–73.

104. Callister TQ, Cooil B, Raya SP, et al. Coronary artery disease: improved reproducibility of calcium scoring with and electron-beam CT volumetric method. Radiology 1998; 208: 807–14.

105. Detrano R, Tang W, Kang X, et al. Accurate coronary calcium phosphate mass measurements from electron beam computed tomograms. Am J Cardiac Imag 1995; 3: 167–73.

106. Becker CR, Kleffel T, Crispin A, et al. Coronary artery calcium measurement: agreement of multirow detector and electron beam CT. Am J Roentgenol 2001; 176: 1295–8.

107. Horiguchi J, Nakanishi T, Ito K. Quantification of coronary artery calcium using multidetector CT and a retrospective ECG-gating reconstruction algorithm. Am J Roentgenol 2001; 177: 1429–35.

108. Knez A, Becker C, Becker A, et al. Determination of coronary calcium with multi-slice spiral computed tomography: a comparitive study with electron-beam CT. Int J Cardiovasc Imag 2002; 18: 295–303.

109. Kopp AF, Ohnesorge B, Becker CR, et al. Reproducibility and accuracy of coronary calcium measurements with multi-detector row versus electron beam CT. Radiology 2002; 225: 113–19.

110. Callister TQ, Cooil B, Raya SP, et al. Coronary artery disease: improved reproducibility of calcium scoring with an electron-beam CT volumetric method. Radiology 1998; 208: 807–14.

111. Ohnesorge B, Kopp AF, Fischbach R, et al. Reproducibility of coronary calcium quantification in repeat examinations with retrospectively ECG-gated multislice spiral CT. Eur Radiol 2002; 12: 1532–40.

112. Takahashi N, Bae KT. Quantification of coronary artery calcium with multi-detector row CT: assessing interscan variability with different tube currents pilot study. Radiology 2003; 228: 101–6.

113. Hong C, Bae KT, Pilgram TK, Zhu F. Coronary artery calcium quantification at multi-detector row CT: influence of heart rate and measurement methods on interacquisition variability initial experience. Radiology 2003; 228: 95–100.

114. Hong C, Becker CR, Schoepf UJ, et al. Coronary artery calcium: absolute quantification in nonenhanced and contrast enhanced multi-detector row CT studies. Radiology 2002; 223: 474–80.

115. Rumberger JA, Simons DB, Fitzpatrick LA, et al. Coronary artery calcium area by electron-beam computed tomography and coronary atherosclerotic plaque area. Circulation 1995; 92: 2157–62.

116. Sangiorgi G, Rumberger JA, Severson A, et al. Arterial calcification and not lumen stenosis is highly correlated with atherosclerotic plaque burden in humans. J Am Coll Cardiol 1998; 31: 126–33.

117. Secci A, Wong N, Tang W, et al. Electron beam computed tomographic coronary calcium as a predictor of coronary events. Circulation 1997; 96: 1122–9.

118. Raggi P, Callister TQ, Cooil B, et al. Identification of patients at increased risk of first unheralded acute myocardial infarction by electron-beam computed tomography. Circulation 2000; 101: 850–5.

119. Callister TQ, Raggi P, Cooil B, et al. Effect of HMG-CoA reductase inhibitors on coronary artery disease by electron-beam computed tomography. N Engl J Med 1998; 339: 1972–8.

120. Achenbach S, Ropers D, Pohle K, et al. Influence of lipid-lowering therapy on the progression of

coronary artery calcification. A prospective evaluation. Circulation 2002; 106: 1077–82.

121. O'Rourke RA, Brundage BH, Froelicher VF, et al. American College of Cardiology/American Heart Association Expert Consensus Document on Electron-Beam Computed Tomography for the Diagnosis and Prognosis of Coronary Artery Disease. Circulation 2000; 102: 126–40.

122. Shaw LJ, Raggi P, Schisterman E, et al. Prognostic value of cardiac risk factors and coronary artery calcium screening for all-cause mortality. Radiology 2003; 228: 826–33.

123. Greenland P, LaBree L, Azen SP, et al. Coronary artery calcium score combined with Framingham score for risk prediction in asymptomatic individuals. J Am Med Assoc 2004; 291: 210–15.

124. Schroeder S, Kopp AF, Baumbach A, et al. Noninvasive detection and evaluation of atherosclerotic coronary plaques with multislice computed tomography. J Am Coll Cardiol 2001; 37: 1430–5.

125. Becker CR, Knez A, Ohnesorge B, et al. Imaging of noncalcified coronary plaques using helical CT with retrospective ECG gating. Am J Roentgenol 2000; 175: 423–4.

126. Kopp AF, Schroeder S, Baumbach A, et al. Noninvasive characterization of coronary lesion morphology and composition by multislice CT: first results in comparison with intracoronary ultrasound. Eur Radiol 2001; 11: 1607–11.

127. Schoenhagen P, Tuzcu EM, Stillman AE, et al. Noninvasive assessment of plaque morphology and remodeling in mildly stenotic coronary segments: comparison of 16-slice computed tomography and intravascular ultrasound. Coron Artery Dis 2003; 14: 459–62.

128. Achenbach S, Moselewski F, Ropers D, et al. Detection of calcified and noncalcified coronary atherosclerotic plaque by contrast-enhanced, submillimeter multidetector spiral computed tomography: a segment-based comparison with intravascular ultrasound. Circulation 2004; 109: 14–17.

129. Schoenhagen P, Ziada KM, Vince DG, et al. Arterial remodeling and coronary artery disease. The concept of 'dilated' versus 'obstructive' coronary atherosclerosis. J Am Coll Cardiol 2001; 38: 297–306.

130. Yamagishi M, Terashima M, Awano K, et al. Morphology of vulnerable coronary plaque: insights from follow-up of patients examined by intravascular ultrasound before and acute coronary syndrome. J Am Coll Cardiol 2000; 35: 106–11.

131. Schoenhagen P, Ziada KM, Kapadia SR, et al. Extent and direction of arterial remodeling in stable versus unstable coronary syndromes: an intravascular ultrasound study. Circulation 2000; 101: 598–603.

132. Mintz GS, Nissen SE, Anderson WD, et al. American College of Cardiology Clinical Expert Consensus Document on Standards for Acquisition, Measurement and Reporting of Intravascular Ultrasound Studies (IVUS). A report of the American College of Cardiology Task Force on Clinical Expert Consensus Documents. J Am Coll Cardiol 2001; 37: 1478–92.

133. Schoenhagen P, Nissen SE. An Atlas and Manual of Coronary Intravascular Ultrasound Imaging. London: Parthenon Publishing, 2004.

134. Achenbach S, Ropers D, Hoffmann U, et al. Assessment of coronary remodeling in stenotic and nonstenotic coronary atherosclerotic lesions by multidetector spiral computed tomography. J Am Coll Cardiol 2004; 43: 842–7.

135. Leber AW, Knez A, Becker A, et al. Accuracy of multidetector spiral computed tomography in identifying and differentiating the composition of coronary atherosclerotic plaques: a comparative study with intracoronary ultrasound. J Am Coll Cardiol 2004; 43: 1241–7.

136. Schroeder S, Flohr T, Kopp AF, et al. Accuracy of density measurements within plaques located in artifical coronary arteries by X-ray multislice CT: results of a phantom study. J Comput Assist Tomogr 2001; 25: 900–6.

137. Schartl M, Bocksch W, Koschyk DH, et al. Use of intravascular ultrasound to compare effects of different strategies of lipid-lowering therapy on plaque volume and composition in patients with coronary artery disease. Circulation 2001; 104: 387–92.

138. Nissen SE, Tuzcu EM, Schoenhagen P, et al.; REVERSAL Investigators. Effect of intensive compared with moderate lipid-lowering therapy on progression of coronary atherosclerosis: a randomized controlled trial. J Am Med Assoc 2004; 291: 1071–80.

139. Nissen SE, Tsunoda T, Tuzcu EM, et al. Effect of recombinant ApoA-I Milano on coronary atherosclerosis in patients with acute coronary syndromes: a randomized controlled trial. J Am Med Assoc 2003; 290: 2292–300.

140. Fayad ZA, Fuster V, Nikolaou K, Becker C. Computed tomography and magnetic resonance imaging for noninvasive coronary angiography and

plaque imaging: current and potential future concepts. Circulation 2002; 106: 2026–34.

141. Yuan C, Mitsumori LM, Ferguson MS, et al. In vivo accuracy of multispectral magnetic resonance imaging for identifying lipid-rich necrotic cores and intraplaque hemorrage in advanced human carotid plaques. Circulation 2001; 104: 2051–6.

142. Rensing BJ, Bongaerts A, van Geuns RJ, et al. Intravenous coronary angiography by electron beam computed tomography: a clinical evaluation. Circulation 1998; 98: 2509–12.

143. Reddy GP, Chernoff DM, Adams JR, Higgins CB. Coronary artery stenoses: assessment with contrast-enhanced electron-beam CT and axial reconstructions. Radiology 1998; 208: 167–72.

144. Budoff MJ, Oudiz RJ, Zalace CP, et al. Intravenous three-dimensional coronary angiography using contrast enhanced electron beam computed tomography. Am J Cardiol 1999; 83: 840–5.

145. Schmermund A, Rensing BJ, Sheddy PF, et al. Intravenous electron-beam computed tomographic coronary angiography for segmental analysis of coronary artery stenoses. J Am Coll Cardiol 1998; 31: 1547–54.

146. Achenbach S, Moshage W, Ropers D, et al. Value of electron-beam computed tomography for the noninvasive detection of high-grade coronary-artery stenoses and occlusions. N Engl J Med 1998; 339: 1964–71.

147. Nieman K, Oudkerk M, Rensing BJ, et al. Coronary angiography with multi-slice computed tomography. Lancet 2001; 357: 599–603.

148. Achenbach S, Giesler T, Ropers D, et al. Detection of coronary artery stenoses by contrast-enhanced, retrospectively electrocardiographically-gated, multislice spiral computed tomography. Circulation 2001; 103: 2535–8.

149. Gerber TC, Kuzo RS, Karstaedt N, et al. Current results and new developments of coronary angiography with use of contrast-enhanced computed tomography of the heart. Mayo Clin Proc 2002; 77: 55–71.

150. Achenbach S, Ropers D, Holle J, et al. In-plane coronary arterial motion velocity: measurement with electron-beam CT. Radiology 2000; 216: 457–63.

151. Schroeder S, Kopp A, Ohnesorge B, et al. Accuracy and reliability of quantitative measurements in coronary arteries by multi-slice computed tomography: experimental and initial clinical results. Clin Radiol 2001; 56: 466–74.

152. Ropers D, Baum U, Pohle K, et al. Detection of coronary artery stenoses with thin-slice multi-detector row spiral computed tomography and multiplanar reconstruction. Circulation 2003; 107: 664–6.

153. Kuettner A, Trabold T, Schroeder S, et al. Noninvasive detection of coronary lesions using 16-detector multislice spiral computed tomography technology – initial clinical results. J Am Coll Cardiol 2004; 44: 1230–37.

154. Fallenberg M, Juergens KU, Wichter T, et al. Coronary artery aneurysm and type-A aortic dissection demonstrated by retrospectively ECG-gate multislice spiral CT. Eur Radiol 2002; 12: 201–4.

155. Engelmann MG, von Smekal A, Knez A, et al. Accuracy of spiral computed tomography for identifying arterial and venous coronary graft patency. Am J Cardiol 1997; 80: 569–74.

156. Dai R, Zhang S, Lu B, et al. Electron-beam CT angiography with three-dimensional reconstruction in the evaluation of coronary artery bypass grafts. Acad Radiol 1998; 5: 863–7.

157. Nieman K, Pattynama PMT, Rensing BJ, et al. Evaluation of patients after coronary artery bypass surgery: CT angiographic assessment of grafts and coronary arteries. Radiology 2003; 229: 749–56.

158. Schlosser T, Konorza T, Hunold P, et al. Noninvasive visualization of coronary artery bypass grafts using 16-detector row computed tomography. J Am Coll Cardiol 2004; 44: 1224–9.

159. Willmann JK, Weishaupt D, Kobza R, et al. Coronary artery bypass grafts: ECG-gated multi-detector row CT angiography – influence of image reconstruction interval on graft visibility. Radiology 2004; 232: 568–77.

160. Gilkeson RC, Markowitz AH, Ciancibello L. Multisection CT evaluation of the reoperative cardiac surgery patient. Recent advances in multi-section CT enable accurate preoperative assessment of patients who have previously undergone cardiac surgery. Radiographics 2003; 23 (Special issue): S3–17.

161. Lu B, Dai R, Bai H, et al. Detection and analysis of intracoronary artery stent after PTCA using contrast-enhanced three-dimensional electron beam tomography. J Invasive Cardiol 2000; 12: 1–6.

162. Maintz D, Grude M, Fallenberg EM, et al. Assessment of coronary arterial stents by multislice-CT angiography. Acta Radiol 2003; 44: 597–603.

163. Schuijf JD, Bax JJ, Jukema JW, et al. Feasibility of assessment of coronary stent patency using 16-slice computed tomography. Am J Cardiol 2004; 94: 427–30.

164. Lawler LP, Corl FM, Fishman EK. Multi-detector row and volume-rendered CT of the normal and accessory flow pathways of the thoracic systemic and pulmonary veins. Radiographics 2002; 22 (Special issue): S45–60.

165. Schaffler GJ, Groell R, Peichel KH, Rienmuller R. Imaging the coronary venous drainage system using electron-beam CT. Surg Radiol Anat 2000; 22: 35–9.

166. Rienmuller R, Groll R, Lipton MJ. CT and MR imaging of pericardial disease. Radiol Clin North Am 2004; 42: 587–601.

167. Axel L. Assessment of pericardial disease by magnetic resonance and computed tomography. J Magn Reson Imag 2004 ; 19: 816–26.

168. Wang ZJ, Reddy GP, Gotway MB, et al. CT and MR imaging of pericardial disease. Radiographics 2003; 23 (Special issue): S167–80.

169. Schwartzman PR, White RD. Imaging of cardiac and paracardiac masses. J Thorac Imag 2000; 15: 265–73.

170. Araoz PA, Mulvagh SL, Tazelaar HD, et al. CT and MR imaging of benign primary cardiac neoplasms with echocardiographic correlation. Radiographics 2000; 20: 1303–19.

171. Sebastià C, Quiroga S, Boyé R, et al. Aortic stenosis: spectrum of diseases depicted at multisection CT. Radiographics 2003; 23 (Special issue): S79–91.

172. White RD, Lipton MJ, Higgins CB, et al. Noninvasive evaluation of suspected thoracic aortic disease by contrast-enhanced computed tomography. Am J Cardiol 1986; 57: 282–90.

173. Castañer E, Andreu M, Gallardo X, et al. CT in nontraumatic acute thoracic aortic disease: typical and atypical features and complications. Radiographics 2003; 23 (Special issue): S93–110.

174. Roos JE, Willmann JK, Weishaupt D, et al. Thoracic aorta: motion artifact reduction with retrospective and prospective electrocardiographic-assisted multidetector row CT. Radiology 2002; 222: 271–7.

175. Flohr T, Prokop M, Becker C, et al. A retrospectively ECG-gated multislice spiral CT scan and reconstruction technique with suppression of heart pulsation artifacts for cardio-thoracic imaging with extended volume coverage. Eur Radiol 2002; 12: 1497–503.

176. Van Arsdell GS, David TE, Butany J. Autopsies in acute type A aortic dissection. Surgical implications. Circulation 1998; 98 (19 Suppl): II299–302.

177. Srichai MB, Lieber ML, Lytle BW, et al. Acute dissection of the descending aorta: noncommunicating versus communicating forms. Ann Thorac Surg 2004; 77: 2012–20.

178. Yoshida S, Akiba H, Tamakawa M, et al. Thoracic involvement of type A aortic dissection and intramural hematoma: diagnostic accuracy – comparison of emergency helical CT and surgical findings. Radiology 2003; 228: 430–5.

179. Coady MA, Rizzo JA, Hammond GL, et al. Penetrating ulcer of the thoracic aorta: what is it? How do we recognize it? How do we manage it? J Vasc Surg 1998; 27: 1006–15.

180. Macleod MR, Amarenco P, Davis SM, Donnan GA. Atheroma of the aortic arch: an important and poorly recognised factor in the aetiology of stroke. Lancet Neurol 2004; 3: 408–14.

181. Watanabe K, Hiroki T, Koga N. Relation of thoracic aorta calcification on computed tomography and coronary risk factors to obstructive coronary artery disease on angiography. Angiology 2003; 54: 433–41.

182. Bortone AS, De Cillis E, D'Agostino D, de Luca Tupputi Schinosa L. Endovascular treatment of thoracic aortic disease: four years of experience. Circulation 2004; 110 (11 Suppl 1): II262–7.

183. Neuhauser B, Perkmann R, Greiner A, et al. Midterm results after endovascular repair of the atherosclerotic descending thoracic aortic aneurysm. Eur J Vasc Endovasc Surg 2004; 28: 146–53.

184. Napoli V, Sardella SG, Bargellini I, et al. Evaluation of the proximal aortic neck enlargement following endovascular repair of abdominal aortic aneurysm: 3-years' experience. Eur Radiol 2003; 13: 1962–71.

185. Schoder M, Cartes-Zumelzu F, Grabenwoger M, et al. Elective endovascular stent-graft repair of atherosclerotic thoracic aortic aneurysms: clinical results and midterm follow-up. Am J Roentgenol 2003; 180: 709–15.

186. Rott A, Boehm T, Soldner J, et al. Computerized modeling based on spiral CT data for noninvasive determination of aortic stent-graft length. J Endovasc Ther 2002; 9: 520–8.

187. MacDonald SL, Mayo JR. Computed tomography of acute pulmonary embolism. Semin Ultrasound CT MR 2003; 24: 217–31.

188. Ruiz Y, Caballero P, Caniego JL, et al. Prospective comparison of helical CT with angiography in

pulmonary embolism: global and selective vascular territory analysis. Interobserver agreement. Eur Radiol 2003; 13: 823–9.

189. van Strijen ME, de Monye W, Kieft GJ, et al. Diagnosis of pulmonary embolism with spiral CT as a second procedure following scintigraphy. Eur Radiol 2003; 13: 1501–7.

190. Carman TL, Deitcher SR. Advances in diagnosis and excluding pulmonary embolism: spiral CT and D-dimer measurement. Cleve Clin J Med 2002; 69: 721–9.

191. Wittram C, Maher MM, Yoo AJ, et al. CT angiography of pulmonary embolism: diagnostic criteria and causes of misdiagnosis. Radiographics 2004; 24: 1219–38.

192. Begemann PG, Bonacker M, Kemper J, et al. Evaluation of the deep venous system in patients with suspected pulmonary embolism with multi-detector CT: a prospective study in comparison to Doppler sonography. J Comput Assist Tomogr 2003; 27: 399–409.

193. Powell T, Muller NL. Imaging of acute pulmonary thromboembolism: should spiral computed tomography replace the ventilation–perfusion scan? Clin Chest Med 2003; 24: 29–38.

194. Lacomis JM, Wigginton W, Fuhrman C, et al. Multi-detector row CT of the left atrium and pulmonary veins before radio-frequency catheter ablation for atrial fibrillation. Radiographics 2003; 23 (Special issue): S35–48.

195. Cronin P, Sneider MB, Kazerooni EA, et al. MDCT of the left atrium and pulmonary veins in planning radiofrequency ablation for atrial fibrillation: a how-to guide. Am J Roentgenol 2004; 183: 767–78.

196. Ghaye B, Szapiro D, Dacher JN, et al. Percutaneous ablation for atrial fibrillation: the role of cross-sectional imaging. Radiographics 2003; 23 (Special issue): S19–33.

197. Saad EB, Marrouche NF, Saad CP, et al. Pulmonary vein stenosis after catheter ablation of atrial fibrillation: emergence of a new clinical syndromes. Ann Intern Med 2003; 138: 634–8.

198. Tatli S, Lipton MJ, Davison BD, et al. MR imaging of aortic and peripheral vascular disease. Radiographics 2003; 23 (Special issue): S59–78.

199. Rubin GD. Techniques for performing multi-detector-row computed tomographic angiography. Tech Vasc Intervent Radiol 2001; 4: 2–14.

200. Tomandl BF, Klotz E, Handschu R, et al. Comprehensive imaging of ischemic stroke with multisection CT. Radiographics 2003; 23: 565–92.

201. Beregi JP, Elkohen M, Deklunder G, et al. Helical CT angiography compared with arteriography in the detection of renal artery stenosis. Am J Roentgenol 1996; 167: 495–501.

202. Castillo M. Diagnosis of disease of the common carotid artery bifurcation: CT angiography vs. catheter angiography. Am J Roentgenol 1993; 161: 395–8.

203. Dillon EH, et al. CT angiography: applications to the evaluation of carotid artery stenosis. Radiology 1993; 189: 211–19.

204. Rubin GD, Schmidt AJ, Logan LJ, Sofilos MC. Multi-detector row CT angiography of lower extremity arterial inflow and runoff: initial experience. Radiology 2001; 221: 146–58.

205. Goo HW, Park IS, Ko JK, et al. CT of congenital heart disease: normal anatomy and typical pathologic conditions. Radiographics 2003; 23: S147–65.

206. Boxt LM. Magnetic resonance and computed tomographic evaluation of congenital heart disease. J Magn Reson Imag 2004; 19: 827–47.

207. Baron MG, Book WM. Congenital heart disease in the adult: 2004. Radiol Clin North Am 2004; 42: 675–90.

208. Ropers D, Moshage W, Daniel WG, et al. Visualization of coronary artery anomalies and their anatomic course by contrast-enhanced electron beam tomography and three-dimensional reconstruction. Am J Cardiol 2001; 87: 193–7.

209. Deibler AR, Kuzo RS, Vohringer M, et al. Imaging of congenital coronary anomalies with multislice computed tomography. Mayo Clin Proc 2004; 79: 1017–23.

210. Azarine A, Lions C, Koussa M, Beregi JP. Rupture of an aneurysm of the coronary sinus of Valsalva: diagnosis by helical CT angiography. Eur Radiol 2001; 11: 1371–3.

211. Hager A, Kaemmerer H, Leppert A, et al. Follow-up of adults with coarctation of the aorta: comparison of helical CT and MRI, and impact on assessing diameter changes. Chest 2004; 126: 1169–76.

Index